A Manual for Differentiation of Bone Marrow-derived Stem Cells to Specific Cell Types

MANUALS IN BIOMEDICAL RESEARCH
ISSN: 1793-1894

Founding Editor: Jan-Thorsten Schantz
(*Technische Universität München, Munich, Germany*)

Series Editor: Ng Kee Woei
(Nanyang Technological University, Singapore)

Published

Forthcoming

Manuals in Biomedical Research – Vol. 8

A Manual for Differentiation of Bone Marrow-derived Stem Cells to Specific Cell Types

Editors

Gilson Khang
Chonbuk National University, Korea

Tatsuya Shimizu
Tokyo Women's Medical University, Japan

Series Editor
Kee Woei Ng

Founding Editor
Jan-Thorsten Schantz

World Scientific

NEW JERSEY · LONDON · SINGAPORE · BEIJING · SHANGHAI · HONG KONG · TAIPEI · CHENNAI

Published by

World Scientific Publishing Co. Pte. Ltd.

5 Toh Tuck Link, Singapore 596224

USA office: 27 Warren Street, Suite 401-402, Hackensack, NJ 07601

UK office: 57 Shelton Street, Covent Garden, London WC2H 9HE

Library of Congress Cataloging-in-Publication Data
A manual for differentiation of bone marrow-derived stem cells to specific cell types /
[edited by] Gilson Khang, Tatsuya Shimizu, Kee Woei Ng.
    p. ; cm. -- (Manuals in biomedical research ; vol. 8)
  Includes bibliographical references and index.
  ISBN 978-9814578233 (pbk. : alk. paper)
  I. Khang, Gilson, editor of compilation. II. Shimizu, Tatsuya, 1968– editor of
compilation. III. Ng, Kee-Woei, editor of compilation. IV. Series: Manuals in
biomedical research ; v. 8.
  [DNLM: 1. Bone Marrow Cells--cytology. 2. Stem Cells--cytology. 3. Tissue
Engineering--methods. WH 380]
  QR185.8.B15
  616.07'98--dc23

                                                        2013041975

British Library Cataloguing-in-Publication Data
A catalogue record for this book is available from the British Library.

Typeset by Stallion Press
Email: enquiries@stallionpress.com

Printed in Singapore by B & Jo Enterprise Pte Ltd

Preface

It has been recognized that tissue engineering and regenerative medicine (TERM) offers an alternative technique to whole organ and tissue transplantation for diseased, failed or malfunctioned organs. The specialty of TERM continues to grow and change rapidly, especially in the stem cell area, which has seen major advances in the last few decades. In terms of academic research and commercialization, this field involves multidisciplinary cooperative works such as adult stem cells, embryonic stem cells and induced pluripotent cells, genetic programming, reprogramming, nuclear transfer, cloning, genomics, proteomics, nanotechnology, biomaterials, and so on.

Thanks to the latest 20 years' endeavor, several stem cell-based therapies are on the boundary of translation from benchside discoveries to clinical therapies. Also, recent intensive works suggest that the use of adult stem cells may not be limited to *in vitro* differentiation for direct cell replacement of damaged tissues. Many works show evidence that adult murine bone marrow cells (BMSCs) possess intrinsic capability to differentiate into adipocytes, osteoblasts, myoblasts, neurons, myoblast, corneal cells, β-cells, chondrocytes, and so on — i.e., they show pluripotent capability. Taken together, it has been reported that BMSCs possess immunosuppressive as well as immunomodulating properties *in vitro* and *in vivo*.

This protocol book is focused on the differentiations of BMSCs into specific cell types that are adapted for the undergraduate and graduate student level. The 19 chapters cover the differentiation methods from conventional small molecules to polymeric scaffolds. We are indebted to the authors for their willing acceptance, devotion and contribution to each recent topic. Also, we very much appreciate the financial support from Chonbuk National University Research Fund in the form of Grants for the Encouragement of Writing. We are truly grateful to the series editor, Jan-Thorsten Schantz and to our publisher, World Scientific Publishing. Also, we would like to give special appreciation to Ms Sook Cheng Lim for her hard work.

Gilson Khang, Ph.D.
Tetsuya Shimizu, Ph.D.
and Kee Woei Ng, Ph.D.

Contents

List of Figures

C

D

F

G

H

K

N

O

R

S

List of Contributors

Hyunhee Ahn
Wake Forest Institute for Regenerative Medicine
Wake Forest School of Medicine
Medicial Center Boulevard
Winston-Salem, NC 27157
USA

Woochul Chang
Cardiovascular Research Institute
Yonsei University College of Medicine
250 Seongsanno, Seodaemun-gu
Seoul, 120-752
Korea

Byung Hyune Choi
Division of Biomedical and Bioengineering Sciences
Inha University College of Medicine
Incheon 400-712
Korea

Jin San Choi
Wake Forest Institute for Regenerative Medicine
Wake Forest School of Medicine
Medical Center Boulevard
Winston-Salem, NC 27157
USA

Kyoung-Hwan Choi
Cell Therapy Center
Department of Orthopedic Surgery and Department
of Molecular Science & Technology
Ajou University, Suwon 442-721
Korea

Rhima M. Coleman
George W. Woodruff School of Mechanical Engineering
Georgia Institute of Technology
801 Ferst Drive, Atlanta, GA 30332
USA
and
Hospital for Special Surgery
535 E. 70th Street
New York, NY 10021
USA

Zigang Ge
Department of Biomedical Engineering
College of Engineering and Center for Biomedical
Materials and Tissue Engineering
Academy for Advanced Interdisciplinary Studies
Peking University
Beijing 100871
China
and
Center for Joint Diseases
Peking University Renmin Hospital
Beijing
P. R. China

Robert E. Guldberg
George W. Woodruff School of Mechanical Engineering
Georgia Institute of Technology
801 Ferst Drive, Atlanta, GA 30332
USA
and
Parker H. Petit Institute for Bioengineering and Bioscience
Georgia Institute of Technology
315 Ferst Drive NW, Atlanta, GA 30332
USA

Ki-Chul Hwang
Cardiovascular Research Institute
Yonsei University College of Medicine
250 Seongsanno, Seodaemun-gu
Seoul, 120-752
Korea

Chun-Ki Joo
Department of Ophthalmology and Visual Science
College of Medicine
The Catholic University of Korea
Gangnam St. Mary Hospital
Korea
505 Banpo-dong
Seocho-gu
Seoul 137-701

Young Min Ju
Wake Forest Institute for Regenerative Medicine
Wake Forest School of Medicine
Medicial Center Boulevard
Winston-Salem, NC 27157
USA

Su Ji Kang
Department of BIN Fusion Tech
Polymer Fusion Res Center & Dept of Polymer Nano Sci Tech
Chonbuk National Univ
567 Baekje-daero, Deokjin
Jeonju 561-756
Korea

Gilson Khang
Department of Polymer Nano Sci & Tech
Department of BIN Fusion Tech and Polymer
Fusion Research Center
Chonbuk National University
567, Beakje-dearo, Deokjin
Jeonju 561-756
Korea

Cho Min Kim
Department of Polymer Nano Sci & Tech
Department of BIN Fusion Tech and Polymer
Fusion Research Center
Chonbuk National University
567, Beakje-dearo, Deokjin
Jeonju 561-756
Korea

Eun Young Kim
Department of Polymer Nano Sci & Tech
Department of BIN Fusion Tech and Polymer
Fusion Research Center
Chonbuk National University
567, Beakje-dearo, Deokjin
Jeonju 561-756
Korea

Jin-Mo Kim
Division of Biomedical and Bioengineering Sciences
Inha University College of Medicine
Incheon 400-712
Korea

Mee-Hae Kim
Department of Biotechnology
Graduate School of Engineering
Osaka University
2-1 Yamadaoka, Suita
Osaka 565-0871
Japan

Shin-Yoon Kim
Department of Orthopaedic Surgery
School of Medicine
Kyungpook National University
Daegu 700-412
Korea

Soon Hee Kim
Department of Polymer Nano Science & Technology
Department of BIN Fusion Tech and Polymer
Fusion Research Center
Chonbuk National University
567, Beakje-dearo, Deokjin
Jeonju 561-756
Korea
and
Cell Therapy Center
Department of Orthopedic Surgery and Department of
Molecular Science & Technology
Ajou University, Suwon 442-721
Korea

Masahiro Kino-oka
Department of Biotechnology
Graduate School of Engineering
Osaka University
2-1 Yamadaoka, Suita
Osaka 565-0871
Japan

Dongwon Lee
Department of Polymer Nano Science & Technology
Department of BIN Fusion Tech and Polymer
Fusion Research Center
Chonbuk National University
567, Beakje-dearo, Deokjin
Jeonju 561-756
Korea

Eun Ah Lee
Musculoskeletal Bioorgan Center
College of Life Sci and Graduate School of Biotech
Kyung Hee Univ
Yongin, Gyeonggi-do, 446-701
Korea

Hyun Jung Lee
Cell Therapy Center
Ajou University
Suwon, 443-270
Korea

Sang Jin Lee
Wake Forest Institute for Regenerative Medicine
Wake Forest School of Medicine
Medical Center Boulevard
Winston-Salem, NC 27157
USA

Yun Mi Lee
Department of BIN Fusion Tech
Polymer Fusion Res Center & Dept of Polymer Nano Sci Tech
Chonbuk National Univ
567 Baekje-daero
Jeonju 561-756

Chao Li
Department of Biomedical Engineering
College of Engineering
Academy for Advanced Interdisciplinary Studies
Peking University
Beijing 100871
China

Jiwon Lim
Department of Pathology and Regenerative Medicine
School of Dentistry
Kyungpook National University
Daegu 700-412
Korea

João F. Mano
3B's Research Group — Biomaterials
Biodegradables and Biomimetics
University of Minho
Headquarters of the European Institute of Excellence
on Tissue Engineering and Regenerative Medicine
AvePark, S. Cláudio de Barco
Caldas das Taipas, Guimarães
Portugal
and
ICVS/3B's — PT Government Associate Laboratory
Braga/Guimarães
Portugal

Byoung-Hyun Min
Cell Therapy Center
Department of Orthopedic Surgery and Department of
Molecular Science & Technology
Ajou University, Suwon 442-721
Korea
and
Cell Therapy Center
Ajou University
Suwon, 443-270
Korea

Hajime Ohgushi
Health Research Institute
National Institute of Advanced Industrial Science and
Technology (AIST)
Osaka
Japan

Joaquim Miguel Oliveira
3B's Research Group — Biomaterials
Biodegradables and Biomimetics
University of Minho
Headquarters of the European Institute of Excellence
on Tissue Engineering and Regenerative Medicine
AvePark, S. Cláudio de Barco
Caldas das Taipas, Guimarães
Portugal
and
ICVS/3B's — PT Government Associate Laboratory
Braga/Guimarães
Portugal

Eui Kyun Park
Department of Pathology and Regenerative Medicine
School of Dentistry
Kyungpook National University
Daegu 700-412
Korea

So Ra Park
Department of Physiology
Inha University College of Medicine
Incheon, 440-712
Korea
and
Division of Biomedical and Bioengineering Sciences
Inha University College of Medicine
Incheon 400-712
Korea

David S. Reece
Wallace H. Coulter Department of Biomedical Engineering
Georgia Institute of Technology and Emory University
313 Ferst Drive, Atlanta, GA 30332
USA

Rui Luís Reis
3B's Research Group — Biomaterials
Biodegradables and Biomimetics
University of Minho
Headquarters of the European Institute of Excellence
on Tissue Engineering and Regenerative Medicine
AvePark, S. Cláudio de Barco
Caldas das Taipas, Guimarães
Portugal
and
ICVS/3B's — PT Government Associate Laboratory
Braga/Guimarães
Portugal

Pamela Gehron Robey
Craniofacial and Skeletal Diseases Branch
National Institute of Dental and Craniofacial Disease
NIH, DHHS, Bethesda
Maryland, 20892
USA

Hong-In Shin
Department of Pathology and Regenerative Medicine
School of Dentistry
Kyungpook National University
Daegu 700-412
Korea

Shay Soker
Wake Forest Institute for Regenerative Medicine
Wake Forest School of Medicine
Medical Center Boulevard
Winston-Salem, NC 27157
USA

Youngsook Son
Musculoskeletal Bioorgan Center
College of Life Sci and Graduate School of Biotech
Kyung Hee Univ
Yongin, Gyeonggi-do, 446-701
Korea

Byeong-Wook Song
Cardiovascular Research Institute
Yonsei University College of Medicine
250 Seongsanno, Seodaemun-gu
Seoul, 120-752
Korea

Jeong Eun Song
Department of Polymer Nano Science & Technology
Department of BIN Fusion Tech and Polymer
Fusion Research Center
Chonbuk National University
567, Beakje-dearo, Deokjin
Jeonju 561-756
Korea

Hazel Y. Stevens
George W. Woodruff School of Mechanical Engineering
Georgia Institute of Technology
801 Ferst Drive, Atlanta, GA 30332
USA

Yasuhiko Tabata
Department of Biomaterials
Institute for Frontier Medical Sciences
Kyoto University
53 Kawara-cho Shogoin
Sakyo-ku, Kyoto 606-8507
Japan

Xiaoyan Tang
Department of Biomedical Engineering
College of Engineering
Academy for Advanced Interdisciplinary Studies
Peking University
Beijing 100871
China

Masaya Yamamoto
Department of Biomaterials
Institute for Frontier Medical Sciences
Kyoto University
53 Kawara-cho Shogoin
Sakyo-ku, Kyoto 606-8507
Japan

Zheng Yang
NUS Tissue Engineering Program
Life Sciences Institute
National University of Singapore
27 Medical Dr,
Singapore 117510
and
Center for Joint Diseases
Peking University Renmin Hospital
Beijing
P. R. China

Hyeon Yoon
Department of BIN Fusion Tech
Polymer Fusion Res Center & Department
of Polymer Nano Sci Tech
Chonbuk National Univ
567 Baekje-daero, Deokjin
Jeonju 561-756
Korea

Introduction

Gilson Khang *

* Dept of Polymer Nano Sci & Tech, Dept of BIN Fusion Tech and Polymer Fusion Research Center, Chonbuk National University, 567, Beakje-dearo, Deokjin, Jeonju 561-756, Korea.

It has been recognized that tissue engineering and regenerative medicine (TERM) offers an alternative technique to whole organ and tissue transplantation for diseased, failed or malfunctioned organs.[1] Millions of patients suffer from end-stage organ failure or tissue loss annually. Recent advances in TERM, including stem cell technology, have shown great potential for clinical trial and research on next-generation medications. Stem cell technology might change the paradigm of the nature of medicine.[2] For example, 18 products were launched in the Korean market after approval from the Korea Food and Drug Administration (KFDA) in 2001, including the world's first autologous bone marrow-derived stem cells (BMSCs) for the treatment of myocardial infarction in 2012, and the world's first allogenic umbilical cord-derived stem cell for the treatment of chondyle defect in the same year. Also, 100 to 200 or more clinical trials (phase I–III) in a broad range of medical areas are in progress throughout the world. Even though this step might be an infant step in the development of regenerative medicine as compared with conventional treatment, it is a good sign for the future use of stem cell therapy.[4]

Adult Stem Cells as Cell Source

To achieve a successful treatment or therapy using regenerative medine technique, a triad of components such as (i) **cells** that are harvested and dissociated from the donor tissue, including nerve, liver, pancreas, cartilage and bone as well as embryonic stem, adult stem or precursor cells; (ii) **biomaterials** such as scaffold substrates to which cells are attached and cultured, resulting in implantation at the desired site of the functioning tissue; and (iii) **growth factors** which promote and/or prevent cell adhesion, proliferation, migration and differentiation by up-regulating or downregulating the synthesis of protein, as well as and receptors, are needed.[1,5]

Among these three basic components, the most critical issue might be the source of the cells. Largely divided, one may consider three general types of stem cell as: (1) embryonic stem cells (ESC); (2) induced pluripotent stem (iPS) cells, including direct reprogramming cells; and (3) adults stem cells. Recently, adult stem cells are extensively applied and tested in research and clinical studies since ESC and iPS can lead to teratoma formation.[2,6] Furthermore, recent studies have shown that some lineage-specific adult stem cells are capable of greater plasticity almost equivalent to ESCs, i.e., the differentiation of mesenchymal stem cell (MSC) can carry out a variety of cell types. For this reason, the plasticity of adult stem cells might be broadened to multipotent, but not pluripotent or totipotent.[7]

Adult stem cells can be derived from every tissue in the body: as bone marrow-derived (BMSC), blood-derived (BSC), adipose-derived (ADSC) as well as umbilical cord blood stem cells (UBMSCs). Also, these adult stem cells can contain hematopoietic stem cells (HSCs), endothelial progenitor cells (EPCs), MSCs, and so on. Each adult stem cell has both advantages and disadvantages in terms of the types of donor and applied injured site. Among these adult stem cells, recently, BMSCs have been receiving attention as the cell source for regenerative medicine because of their capability of differentiation, the ease of manipulation of isolation, the ease of expandability in culture and marker profile.[2,3,7,8]

Readers can find the general introduction to the origin and biology of adult stem cells in textbooks and review papers which have appeared elsewhere.

Importance of Differentiation of BMSC

BMSCs are pluripotent in that they not only act as myelo-regenerative and supportive cells, but can also differentiate into most kinds of cells in our body. For example, HSCs from BMSCs can differentiate into blood cells, bone cells, endothelial cells, including liver cells, skeleton muscle cells, cardiac cells, nerve cells, skin cells, retinal pigment cells and so on.[7] Also, when BMSCs is implanted in *in vivo*, they could help repair multiple tissues blood vessel, heart, liver and so on.[9] This repair has been accomplished in harmony from signaling, mobilization, homing, incorporation, survival, inflammation, proliferation and differentiation of BMSC.[10] It was also followed by a dynamic process of metalloproteinase activity, adhesion molecules and remodeling of extracellular matrix. Among various processes, the differentiation might be the most important for the application of regenerative medicine.[11]

For the differentiation of BMSCs, many methods have been introduced with adjustment to their microenvironment (chemical and physical cues) including chemical induction methods using large or small molecules pellet culture, mechanical stimulation induction methods using cyclic mechano-transduction or ultrasonication, cytokine-released methods using scaffolds, and so on.[12] Until now, chemical cues using soluble factors and substrate coatings have been widely tested and used in maintaining stem cells undifferentiated as well as in accelerating a particular differentiate pathway.[6–8] Of course, extensive references are introduced in so many scientific journals, texts and patents. Recent trends focus on controlling the cellular microenvironment using engineered three-dimensional scaffolds.[11] The protocol methods for the fabrication of scaffolds have already been introduced in the *Book Manuals in Biomedical Research — Vol 4, A Manual for Biomaterials/Scaffold Fabrication Technology*, edited by the author in 2007.[1]

The main aim of this protocol book is to introduce the basic experimental methodology. As we mentioned earlier, many protocols for the differentiation method have appeared in articles, reviews, texts and so on elsewhere.

In Chapters A to F, experimental methods of chondrogenesis of BMSC are introduced: using hydrogel with fibroblast growth factor (FGF) and dexamethasone (Chapter A), alginate macrocapsule loaded with transforming growth factor (TGF-β) (Chapter B), pellet culture (Chapter C), porcine chondrocytes-derived extracellular matrix scaffold (Chapter D), ultrasonication (Chapter E), and chitosan-modified poly(L-lactide-co-ε-caprolactone) scaffolds (Chapter F).

In Chapters G to J, the protocol for osteogenesis of BMSC is introduced: by means of hydroxyapatite/tricalciumphosphate inorganic scaffold with ascorbic acid and dexametasone (Chapter G), dexamethasone-loaded dendrimer nanoparticles onto macroporous hydroxyapatite and starch-polycaprolactone scaffolds (Chapter H), calcium phosphate scaffold with α-ascorbic acid, β-glycerophosphate and dexamethasone (ChapterI) and gelatin and β-tricalciumphosphate scaffolds (Chapter J).

In Chapters K and L, the experimental protocol for cardiomyo-genesisfrom BMSCs is introduced: using dendrimer-immobilized surfaces displaying with D-glucose (Chapter K) and small molecules as protein kinase C (PKC) activator (Chapter L).

The differentiation protocol for differentiation of BMSCs into smooth muscle cells using cocktail medium of TGF-β1 for the application of small diameter vascular graft is described in Chapter M.

From Chapters N to P, the differentiation of BMSCs, into neuronal cell are explained. In Chapter N, the experimental protocol of Schwann cell differentiation of BMSCs by means of the direct co-culture method using insert system is explained. In Chapter O, drug delivery system (DDS) using biodegradable polymers is introduced in the protocol for neurogenesis of BMSC using β-mercaptoethanol released system from β-mercap-toethanol-loaded poly(L-lactide-*co*-glycolide) film. Protocol for neural differentiation from BMSCs using basic fibroblast growth factor (bFGF) and laminin-coating plate is introduced in Chapter P.

From Chapters Q to S, the differentiation of BMSC into eye-related cells is shown. In Chapter Q, the protocol for differentia-tion of retinal pigment epithelial-like cells from BMSCs using co-culture method is introduced. The experimental protocol for differentiation of olfactory ensheathing cells from BMSCs by insertion and conditioned media system is introduced in Chapter R. Finally, Chapter S introduces the protocol for the differentiation of BMSCs into corneal endothelial cells by direct and indirect co-culture.

Summary

The main aim of this protocol book is the introduction of basic experimental methods for the differentiation of BMSCs to stu-dents and scientists in the academia and industry in stem cell engineering fields. In the 19 chapters, we show very few spe-cific cell types, very few scaffolds, very few chemical cues as well as microenvironments as compared with very recent mas-sive works for the development of differentiation methods of

BMSCs for application in regenerative medicine. However, despite these limited chapters, we tried to introduce the basic experimental methods, including characterization assay methods and the importance of differentiation of BMSCs as much as we can. As discussed earlier, more detailed experimental methods and another methodology for the differentiation of BMSCs can be found elsewhere.

Editing of successive books on other differentiation protocols for adipocyte-derived stem cell, umbilical cord blood-derived stem cell and so on is now in progress.

Acknowledgments

This research was supported by WCU (R31-20029, KMEST), Bio-industry Technology Development Program (112007-05-1-SB010, MKFAFF), Bio & Medical Technology Development Program (2012M3A9C6050204, KMEST) and Chonbuk National University Research Fund as Grants for the Encouragement of Writing.

References

1. G Khang, MS Kim, HB Lee. (2007) *Manuals in Biomedical Research Vol 4, A Manual for Biomaterials/Scaffold Fabrication Technology*, World Scientific, Singapore.
2. RM Nerem. (2011) Chapter 1, Tissue Engineering: From Basic Biology to Cell-Based Applications. In: S Li, N L'Heureux, J Elisseett (eds), *Stem Cell and Tissue Engineering*, World Scientific, Singapore, pp. 1–11.
3. G Khang. (2012) Importance of inflammation reaction of scaffold for the application of regenerative medicine. *Inflammation and Regeneration* **32**(5): 178.
4. MJ Lysaght, A Jaklence, E Deweerd. (2008) Great expectation: Private sector activity in tissue engineering, regenerative medicine and stem cell therapies. *Tissue Eng, Part* A **14**(2): 305.
5. G Khang, SH Kim, MS Kim, HB Lee. (2008) Hybrid, Composite, and Complex Biomaterials for Scaffolds. In: R Lanza, A Atala, R Nerem, W Thomson (eds), *Principles of Regenerative Medicine*, Academic Press, New York, pp. 636–655.

6. ME Furth, A Atala. (2008) Chapter 1, Current and Future Perspectives of Regenerative Medicine. In: Ref [5], pp. 2–15.

7. RG Edward. (2004) Stem cells to today: Bone marrow stem cells. *Reprod Biomed* **9**: 541.

8. T Ahsan, AM Doyle, RM Nerem. (2008) Chapter 3, Stem Cell. Research. In: Ref [5], pp. 28–47.

9. MF Pettinger, BJ Martin. (2004) Mesenchymal stem cells and their potential as cardiac therapeutics. *Circ Res* **95**: 9.

10. M Xaymardan, M Cimni, RD Weisel, R-K Li. (2008) Chapter 16, Bone Marrow Stem Cells: Properties and Pluripotency. In: Ref [5], pp. 268–283.

11. G Khang. (2012) Chapter 1, Introduction. In: G Khang (ed), *Handbook of Intelligent Scaffold for Tissue Engineering & Regenerative Medicine*, Pan Stanford Pub, New York, pp. 3–40.

12. DE Disher, DJ Mooney, PW Zandstra. (2009) Growth factors, matrices and forces combine and control stem cells. *Science* **324**: 1673.

A

Chondrogenic Differentiation of Rat BMSCs in Hydrogel

Hazel Y. Stevens*,
David S. Reece[†],
Rhima M. Coleman*,[‡] and
Robert E. Guldberg*,[§]

* George W. Woodruff School of Mechanical Engineering, Georgia Institute of Technology, 801 Ferst Drive, Atlanta, GA 30332.

[†] Wallace H. Coulter Department of Biomedical Engineering, Georgia Institute of Technology and Emory University, 313 Ferst Drive, Atlanta, GA 30332.

[‡] Hospital for Special Surgery, 535 E. 70th Street, New York, NY 10021.

[§] Parker H. Petit Institute for Bioengineering and Bioscience, Georgia Institute of Technology, 315 Ferst Drive NW, Atlanta, GA 30332, USA.

Background

- Cartilage has a low capacity for self repair. Autologous tissue engineering strategies are limited by the difficulty in obtaining sufficient cells without causing further injury. Moreover, *in vitro* expansion of chondrocytes to increase cell yield causes dedifferentiation, with an associated decreased expression of type II collagen and sulfated glycosaminoglycans (sGAGs) and an increased expression of type I collagen.

- Bone marrow-derived mesenchymal stromal cells (BMSCs) show promise as an alternative cell source by virtue of the fact that they can undergo chondrogenesis in high density monolayer in the presence of growth factors such as transforming growth factor (TGF-β1), fibroblast growth factor-2 (FGF-2) or dexamethasone (Dex). However, the recovery and maintenance of the chondrocytic phenotype is better achieved by growth in 3D culture systems.

- Encapsulation of BMSCs in 3D hydrogels such as alginate and agarose mimics the extracellular matrix environment[1,2] and ensures adequate mass transfer of gases and nutrients. As gels can be injected and polymerized *in situ,* the technique lends itself to arthroscopic repair of cartilaginous lesions.

- Culture of BMSCs in pellets is an alternative 3D culture system and is "scaffold-free." This environment allows for cell-to-cell contact and mass transfer gradients similar to stages of embryonic cartilage and bone development.

- Mesenchymal stem cells can also be derived from human and rodent amniotic fluid and these amniotic fluid-derived stem (AFS) cells are a putative source for large numbers of chondroprogenitor cells.

- We investigated the effects of 3D culture systems on the response of rat BMSCs (rBMSCs)[1] and human AFS (hAFS)[2] cells to chondrogenic growth factors.

Isolation and 2D Expansion of rBMSCs

- Excise femurs and tibiae from Sprague-Dawley rats and remove the growth plates from proximal and distal ends using a bone cutter.

- Use a 20 gauge needle attached to a 10 mL syringe to flush the marrow cavity with α-MEM containing FBS and 1% antibiotics (100 U/mL penicillin and 100 µg/mL streptomycin).
- Centrifuge at 1200 rpm for 20 min, resuspend in media and plate at 1 leg/100 mm diameter dish for 30 min.
- Collect media containing unattached cells, spin down and replate at a density of 150×10^6 cells/T-150 flask. Incubate for 8 days with a media change at 4 days.
- Trypsinize confluent cultures at day 8 (Passage 0), replate at 1×10^6 cells/T-150 flask and grow to confluence (P1). Repeat this process thrice to reach P4.
- Treat monolayers with 1 ng/mL recombinant human FGF-2 from P1 to P4.

Hydrogel Encapsulation for 3D Culture

- Prepare 2% solutions of sodium alginate or agarose type VII using Ca^{2+}/Mg^{2+} free PBS. Autoclave for 20 min to dissolve the powder and sterilize the solutions.
- Pre-wet cellulose-acetate membrane with 102 mM $CaCl_2$, 100 mM NaCl and 50 mM HEPES to cross-link alginate gels or with PBS to support agarose gels. Suspend cells in the hydrogel solution at 20×10^6/mL and pipette ≈25 uL into the well of a custom-designed mold (Fig. 1). Allow to polymerize for 30 min at RT. Wells are 4–8 mm diameter and 2 mm thick.
- Rinse gels in media with antibiotics and culture released gels in a 24 well plate in 1–2 mL basal media at 37°C, 5% CO_2 in a humidified atmosphere.
- Basal media is DMEM with 1% ITS+ (BD), 1% antibiotic, antimycotic (0.025 µg/mL amphotericin), 0.1 mM non-essential amino acids and 50 µg/mL ascorbic acid-2-phosphate (AA2P). Change media every 2–3 days. Chondrogenic media includes basal media plus supplements such as 10 nM Dex or 10 ng/mL TGF-β1 + 10 nM Dex (Fig. 2).

Pellet Culture

- Harvest cells at 70% confluency. Seed 200 000 cells into each 15 mL conical tube in basal or chondrogenic media.

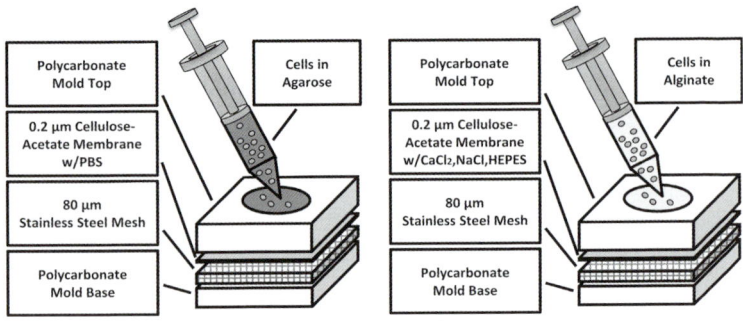

Fig. 1 Cartoon of process of injecting cells and hydrogel into the custom-designed mold.

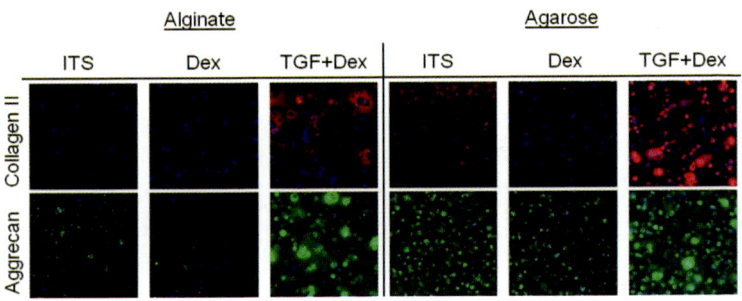

Fig. 2 Collagen type II (red) and aggrecan (green) immunolocalization in hydrogels at 21 days in culture. Cells were treated with FGF-2 during monolayer expansion and ITS, Dex or TGF-β1+Dex during 3D culture.

For this culture, basal media is DMEM supplemented with 1% ITS+, 1% antibiotics, 2 mM L-glutamine, 100 nM Dex, 40 μg/mL L-proline, and 50 μg/mL AA2P. Chondrogenic media is basal media plus either 10 ng/mL TGF-β3, 10 ng/mL TGF-β3 with 500 ng/mL BMP-2 or 10 ng/mL TGF-β1.

- Centrifuge tubes for 5 min at 500 g to condense the cells. Cells form pellets within 24 hrs. Culture pellets in 0.5 mL media, 37°C, 5% CO_2. Change media every 3–4 days for 3 weeks. Pellet sizes resulting from culture in different chondrogenic media are shown in Fig. 3.

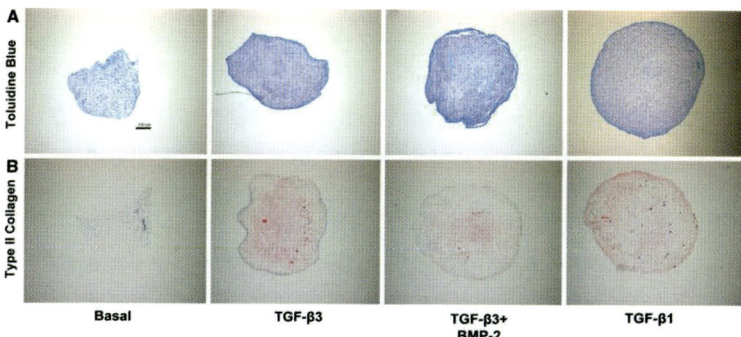

Fig. 3 Chondrogenic differentiation of hAFS cells in pellet culture. (A) Size and sGAG (stains purple with toluidine blue) amount is growth factor dependent. (B) Collagen type II immunolocalization detected by red coloration. Scale bar is 100 μm and applies to all images.

Assessment of Chondrogenesis and Cell Viability

- sGAG content measured by DMMB assay.
- DNA content measured by Hoechst 33258 dye.
- Immunolocalization of cartilage specific collagen type II and aggrecan by confocal microscopy and nuclear counterstain.
- Cell viability using Live/Dead Assay (Invitrogen).

Requirements

Sprague-Dawley rat femurs, custom mold with cellulose acetate membrane, Minimum Essential Medium Eagle Alpha Modification (α-MEM), Dulbecco's modified Eagle's medium (DMEM), 1% antibiotics (100 unit/mL penicillin and 100 μg/mL streptomycin), ITS+, amphotericin, non-essential amino acids, PBS, ascorbic acid-2-phosphate, L-proline, L-glutamine, Dex, 0.05% trypsin-EDTA, FBS, Pronova UP LVG sodium alginate, agarose type VII, CaCl$_2$, NaCl, HEPES, growth factors, hAFS cells (c-kit positive), DMMB assay, Hoechst 33258 dye, antibodies, Live/Dead Assay, 20 gauge needle, cell culture dishes.

Characterization

- rBMSCs expanded to P2 with FGF-2 1 ng/mL supplementation, encapsulated in alginate and exposed to TGF-β1 10 ng/mL + Dex 10 nM showed the greatest sGAG content per cell at 21 days (Fig. 4).

- In agarose, highest sGAG/DNA values were achieved when rBMSCs were expanded without FGF-2 but given TGF-β1 + Dex after encapsulation (Fig. 4). However, recent studies suggest that pre-differentiation of rBMSCs, before agarose encapsulation and delivery to rat growth plate defects, negatively impacted their therapeutic potential.[3]

- The addition of growth factors to the media after encapsulation decreased rBMSC viability in both alginate and agarose gels, with the agarose gels showing the most cell death (Fig. 5).

- Comparison of hBMSC and hAFS sGAG/DNA levels suggests that the chondrogenic differentiation capability of hBMSCs far exceeds that of hAFS cells under these culture conditions (Fig. 6). Cell number and sGAG/DNA levels of hAFS cell pellet cultures were not significantly affected by FGF-2 supplementation (Fig. 6).

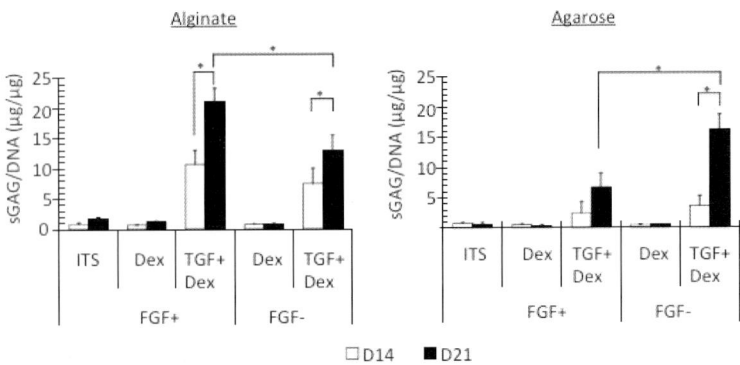

Fig. 4 rBMSCs expanded to P2 ± FGF-2 and encapsulated in alginate or agarose and cultured for 14 and 21 days. sGAG normalized to total DNA.

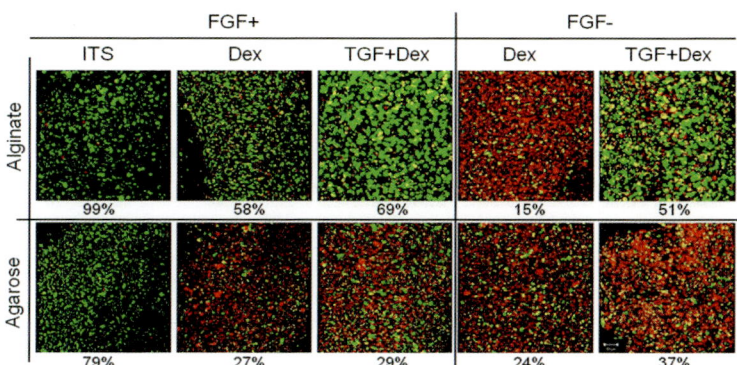

Fig. 5 Live–dead staining of alginate and agarose gels after 21 days of culture. Original magnification was ×10. Live and dead cells fluoresce green and red, respectively.

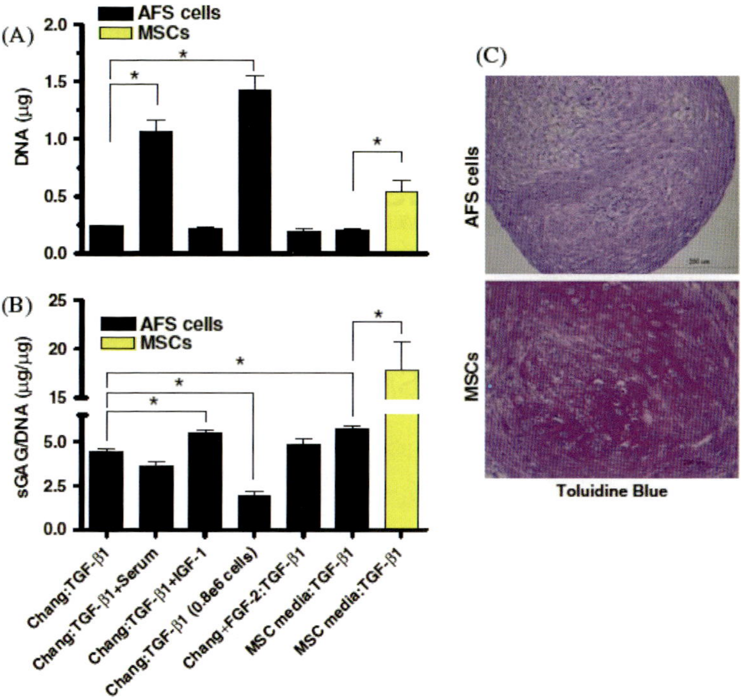

Fig. 6 Pellet culture. DNA content (A) and sGAG normalized to DNA content for hAFS cells and hBMSCs grown first in expansion media, then later in pellet culture with supplements listed (B). sGAG staining for hBMSC vs. smaller hAFS cell pellets (C).

Notes

- An alternative to the $CaCl_2$ wetted membrane is $CaSO_4$ (8.4 μg/mL) premixing via a syringe connector. Gels pre-formed in the syringe have greater porosity when delivered but less mechanical integrity.
- Agarose gels do not need any cross-linker for polymerization as they rely on the cooling step. They must be injected immediately to prevent gelling in the syringe.
- Prior to immunohistochemical staining of alginate, treat the gels with barium chloride for 30 min under agitation for permanent crosslinking. Use 0.01% Triton-X and 0.05 U/mL chondroitinase pre-treatments before aggrecan and collagen type II immunostaining.
- hAFS were expanded in Chang media before being harvested and cultured as pellets. Chang media is α-MEM with 16% FBS, 1% antibiotics, 2 mM L-glutamine, 18% Chang B and 2% Chang C (Irvine Scientific) supplements.

References

1. RM Coleman, ND Case, RE Guldberg. (2007) Hydrogel effects on bone marrow stromal cell response to chondrogenic growth factors. *Biomaterials* **28**: 2077–2086.
2. YM Kolambkar, A Peister, S Soker, *et al.* (2007) Chondrogenic differentiation of amniotic fluid-derived stem cells. *J Mol Hist* **38**: 405–413.
3. RM Coleman, Z Schwartz, BD Boyan, RE Guldberg. (2012) The therapeutic effect of bone marrow-derived stem cell implantation after epiphyseal plate injury is abrogated by chondrogenic predifferentiation. *Tissue Engineering, Part A* Oct 10, 2012 epub.

B

Protocol of Chondrogenesis from BMSCs using TGF-β Loaded Alginate Bead

Soon Hee Kim and Gilson Khang

Background

- Natural cartilage tissue has limited self-repair capability. Autologous transplant causes donor-site morbidity and cell dedifferentiation. Therefore, the cartilage tissue engineering field has focused on mesenchymal stem cell (MSCs) as an alternative cell source

Dept of PolymerNano Sci & Tech, Dept of BIN Fusion Tech and Polymer Fusion Research Center, Chonbuk National University, 567, Beakje-dearo, Deokjin, Jeonju 561-756, Korea.

because MSCs can be differentiated to chondrocytes under proper stimulation and are easier to obtain. They also have much higher cell proliferation.

- MSCs derived from bone marrow (BMSCs) of these organs can be easily obtained by bone marrow suction and expanded over several subcultures maintaining their ability of differentiation.

- Bone morphogenic proteins as TGF-β superfamily can further stimulate chondrogenesis. TGF-β1 is the most commonly used growth factor for chondrogenesis of MSC and that has been shown to stimulate chondrocyte proteoglycan synthesis and the amounts of collagen type II and proteoglycans in MSCs *in vitro*. In addition, production of sulfated glycosaminoglycan (sGAG) and type II collagen was increased more by TGF-β1 than by TGF-β3.

- It has been known that scaffolds play an important role in cartilage regeneration. If chondrocytes are cultured under two-dimensional conditions, they start to dedifferentiate and to lose their chondrogenic phenotype and activity while when culturing under three-dimensional conditions, they recover a chondrogenic phenotype related with redifferentiation process.

- We introduced the chondrogenesis of BMSCs using TGF-β1 loaded alginate beads by mixing BMSCs.

Culturing Methods of BMSCs

- Isolate femurs (or tibias) from Fischer rat legs and wash them with PBS.

- Flush the marrow cavity with 1 mL of PBS using 26 gauge syringes into tube with PBS.

- Layer marrow onto a Percoll cushion and centrifuge obtained marrow for 5 min at 2000 rpm.

- Maintain the resulting BMSC suspension in a humidified atmosphere of 5% CO_2 at 37°C and culture them with DMEM including 10% FBS and 1% antibiotics in culture flask at a density of 10^3–10^4 cell/cm^2.

- Remove the non-adherent hematopoietic cells after three days by washing with PBS including antibiotics, and culture the adherent spindle-shaped BMSCs for 10 days. The medium was changed every 2–3 days.

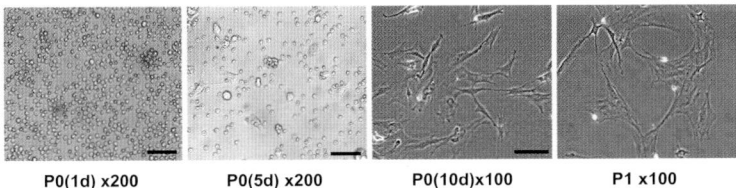

P0(1d) x200   P0(5d) x200   P0(10d)x100   P1 x100

Fig. 1 BMSC morphology from primary culture to passage 1 (P: passage, scale bar: 250 µm in magnification ×100, 100 µm in magnification ×200).[2]

- Subculture when these primary BMSCs reach 80–90% of confluence, and use the BMSCs passage 2 or 3 times.
- Isolated BMSCs showed fibroblast-like morphology (Fig. 1).

BMSC Characterization

- Analyze properties of MSC in isolated BMSCs by immunocytochemistry or FACS using four antibodies at least.
- BMSCs were lacking CD45- and CD34- as hematopoietic stem cell markers whereas they were positively stained CD29- and CD44- through IHC (Fig. 2).

Preparation of Alginate Beads[1]

- Sterilize low viscosity sodium alginate by UV illumination overnight.
- Dissolve sterilized sodium alginate at 1.2% (w/v) in a filtrated PBS.
- Mix TGF-β1 of 0.5 µg/mL and 0.1 mg/mL heparin (heparin stabilizes TGF-β1 release by difference of concentration of inside and outside gel) in an alginate solution.
- Resuspend BMSCs in alginate solution at 3×10^5 cells/mL.
- Gently mix the cell suspension and then drop through a 23 gauge syringe needle into 102 mM $CaCl_2$ solution.
- Put the beads in a $CaCl_2$ solution for 10 min to allow absolute cross-linking reaction.
- Wash the beads three times with PBS.

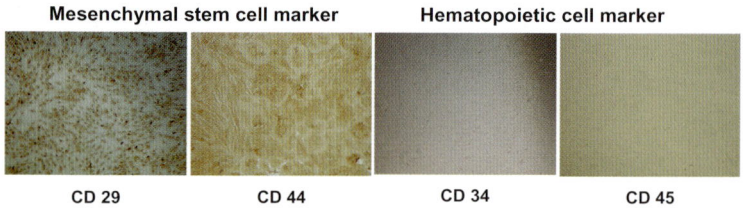

Mesenchymal stem cell marker **Hematopoietic cell marker**

CD 29   CD 44   CD 34   CD 45

Fig. 2   Confirmation of mesenchymal stem cell marker in cultured BMSCs.

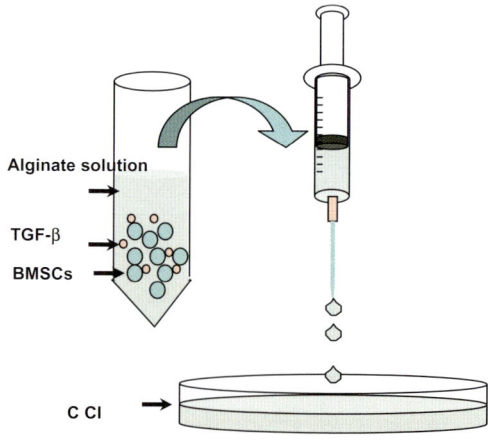

Fig. 3   Schematic representation of process of preparing alginate bead. The concentration of TGF-β1: 0.5 µg/mL, alginate solution: 1.2 w/v%, CaCl$_2$: 102 mM.[2]

- When drops of an alginate solution are put into a CaCl$_2$ solution containing divalent metal ions, soluble alginate chains immediately formed sphere-shaped bead cross-linking by calcium chloride (Fig. 3).
- 100 beads were fabricated per alginate solution of 1 mL; average diameter was about 2.5 mm and the gross morphology is sphere-like.
- Alginate bead successfully encapsulated BMSCs (Fig. 4).

Analysis for Chondrogenesis *In Vitro* and *In Vivo*

- DMMB assay for sulfated GAG contents
- Hydroxyproline assay for collagen contents

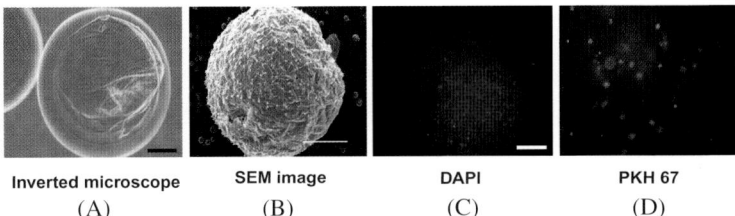

Inverted microscope	SEM image	DAPI	PKH 67
(A)	(B)	(C)	(D)

Fig. 4 (A, B) The observation of empty beads by inverted microscope and SEM. (C) Fluorescence microscope of alginate beads including BMSCs and TGF-β1 (scale bar: 500 μm in magnification ×40).[2]

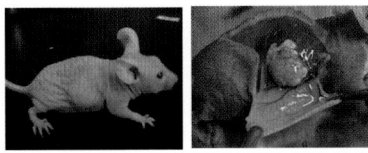

Fig. 5 Gross morphology after extracting subcutaneous implanted alginate bead.[2]

- Lacunae observation as evidence of chondrocyte by histology
- Collagen type II which mainly found chondrocyte and exists in cells or around cells and collagen type I confirmation as dedifferentiation marker by immunohistochemistry (IHC)
- Safranin-O or alcian blue staining for proteoglycan
- RT-PCR for collagen type I and II and aggrecan
- If you need to do analysis *in vivo*, implant beads into the back of BALB/c-nu nude mouse. Mix 200 μL 20 w/v% of Pluronic F127 with beads of 40–50 to inhibit the spread of beads in *in vivo* environment. And evaluate in the same method with *in vitro* analysis (Fig. 5).

Requirements

Dulbecco's modified Eagle's medium (DMEM, low glucose), antibiotics (100 unit/mL penicillin and 100 μg/mL streptomycin), PBS, trypsin-EDTA, FBS, low viscosity (250 cps in 2% solution at 25°C) sodium alginate, calcium chloride, heparin (optional), TGF-β1, syringe (23 gauge) and needed cell culture wares.

Characterization

- Alginate beads including BMSCs and TGF-β1 formed cartilaginous tissues that were similar to the native cartilage, as evidenced by chondrocytes within lacunae during implantation time (Fig. 6).
- Through results of Safranin-O and Alcian Blue staining, blue and red color consistent with the presence of GAG and proteoglycan, respectively, was found within the lacunae of the experimental specimen. The color generally has become denser with time (Fig. 7).
- We could observe positive expression for type II collagen in the beads. The intensity of type II collagen in bead appeared somewhat higher in 4 and 6 weeks than in 2 weeks (Fig. 7).
- These results could demonstrate that the synergistic effects of mixing TGF-β1 and BMSCs induced chondrogenesis of BMSCs in alginate bead.

Notes

- It is possible to add ascorbate 2-phosphate or dexamethasone during cultivation to enhance chondrogenesis.
- Bead size can be controlled by dropping rate and the size of syringe gauge.
- If you transplant many beads into a body, take care for beads mass not to be thickened for sufficient nutrient supply.

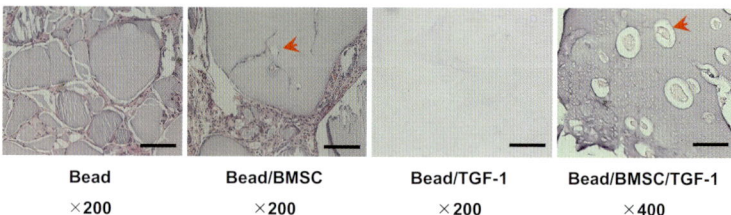

| Bead | Bead/BMSC | Bead/TGF-1 | Bead/BMSC/TGF-1 |
| ×200 | ×200 | ×200 | ×400 |

Fig. 6 Photomicrographs from H&E histological sections of alginate beads implanted for 4 weeks (scale bar: 100 μm in magnification ×200, 50 μm in magnification × 400).[2]

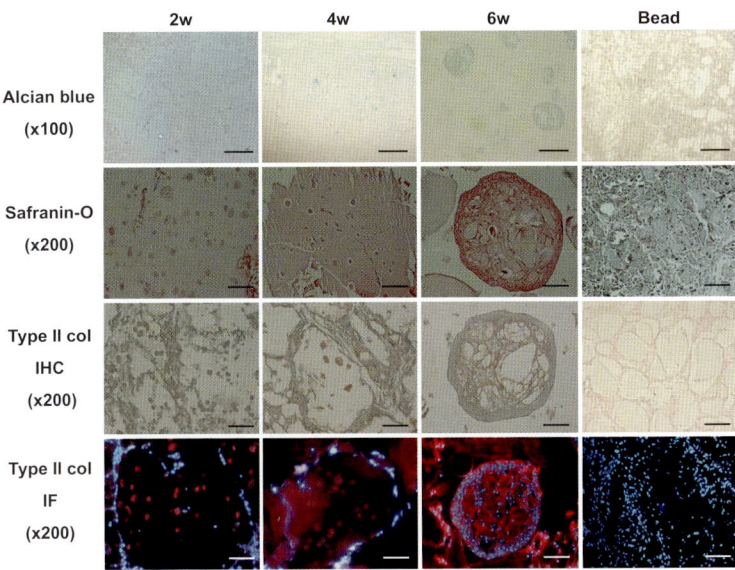

Fig. 7 Alcian Blue staining, Safranin-O staining, and IHC and immunofluorescence (IF) for type II collagen in beads including BMSCs and TGF-β1 (scale bar: 250 μm for magnification ×100 and 100 μm for magnification ×200).

- Remove factors that affect the results in analysis (for example, remove alginate in Safranin-O or Alcian Blue staining, then we may obtain clear results).

Acknowledgments

This research was supported by WCU (R31-20029, KMEST), Bio-industry Technology Development Program (112007-05-1-SB010, MKFAFF) and Bio & Medical Technology Development Program (2012M3A9C6050204, KMEST).

References

1. KS Park, CM Jin, SH Kim, *et al.* (2005) Chondrogenic differentiation of bone marrow stromal cells in transforming growth factor-β1 loaded alginate bead. *Macromolecular Res* **13**(4): 285–292.

2. SM Kim, JW Jang, SH Jung, *et al.* (2008) Chondrogenesis of rat bone marrow stromal cells in Transforming growth factor-β1 loaded alginate bead *in vivo*. *Tissue Eng Regen Med* **5**(4): 650–659.

C

Protocol of Chondrogenesis from Human BMSCs by Pellet Culture

Jeong Eun Song, Eun Young Kim, Soon Hee Kim and Gilson Khang

Dept of PolymerNano Sci & Tech, Dept of BIN Fusion Tech and Polymer Fusion Research Center, Chonbuk National University, 567 Beakje-daero, Deokjin, Jeonju 561-756, Korea.

Background

- It is well known that damaged articular cartilage has a limited potential for repair or regeneration due to avascularity and the presence of relatively few cells with low mitotic activity.
- MSCs can be isolated easily, expanded in culture, and stimulated to differentiate into bone, cartilage, neuron, muscle, marrow stroma, tendon, fat and a variety of other connective tissues.
- BMSCs may represent a convenient source of stem cells for cell-mediated gene therapy and tissue engineering applications. BMSCs exhibit self-renewal capabilities and multipotentiality. The human bone marrow contains MSCs capable of differentiating along multiple mesenchymal cell lineages.
- We will introduce a culture system that is a reliable and reproducible for successful *in vitro* chondrogenesis of human BMSCs. We used both pellet culture and proper differentiation medium to provide environment similar with *in vivo*.

Culturing Methods of Human BMSCs

- Obtain bone marrow from iliac crest of human donors (age range: 18–38 years) (Fig. 1).
- Mix 25 mL of heparinized bone marrow (6000 unit heparin) with an equal volume of serum-free low glucose-DMEM medium supplemented with an antibiotic-antimycotic solution (100 U/mL penicillin G, 100 μg/mL streptomycin, 250 ng/mL amphotericin B).
- Slowly add marrow onto a 50% Percoll cushion, after which centrifuge it at 2500 rpm for 25 min in order to isolate stromal cells.
- Extract nucleated cells in the middle layer, wash in PBS, and centrifuge at 1000 rpm for 10 min (Fig. 2).
- Re-suspend cell pellet obtained from adult bone marrow in BMSC culture medium which consists of DMEM containing 10% FBS and 1% antibiotic-antimycotic solution.

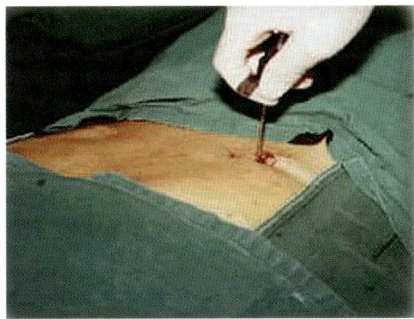

Fig. 1 Bone marrow aspiration from human iliac crest.[1]

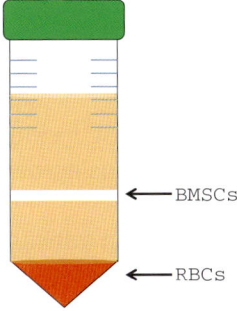

Fig. 2 Percoll gradient centrifugation of human BMSC (RBCs: red blood cells).[1]

- Plate at 10^3–10^4 cells/cm^2 in tissue-cultured flasks and maintain cultures at 37°C in a humidified atmosphere containing 5% CO_2.
- Change the medium every 2–3 days.
- Harvest cells by treatment with trypsin when primary hBMSCs reach 80–90% of confluence. Use hBMSCs within passages 3–5 at the time of the experiment.

hBMSC Characterization

- Isolated human BMSCs showed fibroblast-like morphology (Fig. 3).

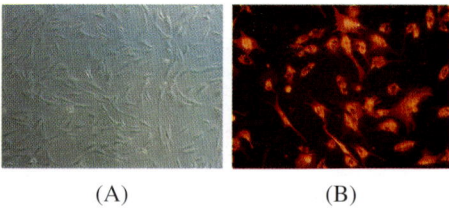

(A)   (B)

Fig. 3   Primary culture of human BMSCs for 5 days. (A) Cell morphology using reverse phase microscope (magnification ×50), (B) cell morphology using red cell tracer (magnification ×100).

Chondrogenesis from hBMSC by Pellet Culture

- Harvest cells within passages 3–5 using trypsin-EDTA.
- Spin down detached cells at 1200 rpm for 3 min in 50 mL polypropylene conical tubes.
- Re-suspend with human BMSC culture medium, count cell number at 1×10^6 cells/mL using hemocytometer and add them to 15 mL conical tube.
- Treat 1 mL of culture medium which consists of serum-free high glucose (4.5 g/L) DMEM supplemented with 10 ng/mL TGF-β3, 100 nM dexamethasone, 50 μg/mL ascorbic acid, 1.24 mg/mL bovine serum albumin, 100 μg/mL sodium pyruvate and 40 μg/mL L-proline. Incubate cell pellet at 37°C in a humidified atmosphere containing 5% CO_2.
- Change medium every 2 days.
- On culture day 14, replace above mentioned medium with new medium, consisting of high glucose (4.5 g/L) DMEM supplemented with 50 nM thyroxine, 20 mM β-glycerophosphate, 1 nM dexamethasone, 50 μg/mL ascorbic acid, 1.24 mg/mL bovine serum albumin, 100 μg/mL sodium pyruvate and 40 μg/mL L-proline (Fig. 4).

Available Analysis for Chondrogenesis of Human BMSCs

- DMMB assay for sulfated GAG contents.
- Hydroxyproline assay for collagen contents.
- Lacunae observation as evidence of chondrocyte by histology.

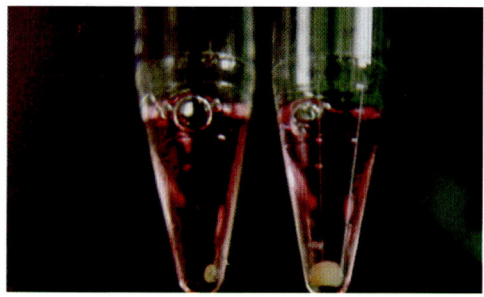

Fig. 4 Differentiation of human BMSCs by pellet culture system. Cell pellet was maintained in differentiation medium.[1]

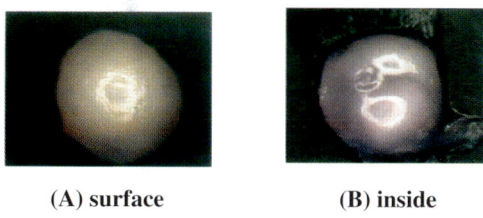

| **(A) surface** | **(B) inside** |

Fig. 5 Confirmation of pellet morphology by hi-scope.[2]

- Collagen type II which mainly found chondrocyte and exists in cells or around cells and collagen type I confirmation as dedifferentiation marker by immunohistochemistry (IHC).
- Safranin-O or Alcian Blue staining for proteoglycan.
- RT-PCR for collagen type I and II and aggrecan.

Characterization

- Cell pellets that were differentiated by pellet culture system and chondrogenesis medium exhibited smooth and glistening morphology as normal cartilage (Fig. 5).
- Cells were strongly aggregated in cell pellet (Fig. 6). Pellet culture system allows cell–cell interactions analogous to those that occur in precartilage condensation during embryonic development.
- After 14 days of culture, pellet maintained in high-glucose medium with 10 ng/mL TGF-β3 stained with Safranin-O

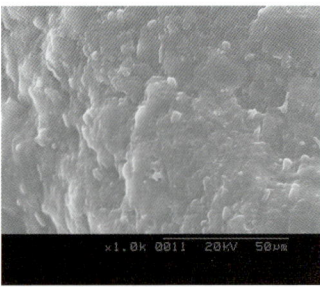

Fig. 6 SEM picture of cell pellet (magnification ×1000).[2]

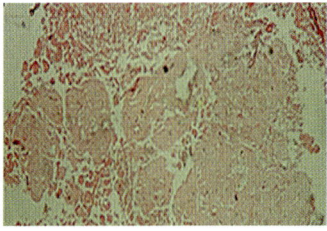

Fig. 7 Safranin-O staining of human BMSCs cultured as aggregates. (magnification ×200).[1]

(Fig. 7). This means that human BMSCs cultured as aggregates synthesized proteoglycan.

Requirements

DMEM (low glucose and high glucose), TGF-β3, dexamethasone, ascorbic acid, bovine serum albumin, sodium pyruvate, L-proline, thyroxine, β-glycerophosphate, antibiotic-antimycotic solution, PBS, trypsin-EDTA, FBS, conical tube (15 mL and 50 mL), centrifuge and other instruments for cell culture.

Notes

• It should be tested that cultured human BMSCs are uniformly positive for CD29, CD44 and negative for hematopoietic markers CD34 and CD45 by flow cytometry or immunocytochemistry.

- Pellet culture without treatment of differentiation medium could not be sufficient for the induction of chondrogenesis due to absence of bioactive factors.

Acknowledgments

This research was supported by WCU (R312-0029, KMEST), Bio-industry Technology Development Program (112007-05-1-SB010, MKFAFF) and Bio & Medical Technology Development Program (2012M3A9C6050204, KMEST).

References

1. HJ Hwang, G Khang, JH Sung, *et al.* (2002) Chondrogenic differentiation from bone marrow-derived mesenchymal stem cell by pellet culture: Preliminary study. *Biomaterials Research* **6**(2): 45–52.

2. KS Park, EJ Kim, G Khang, *et al.* (2003) Chondrogeneic differentiation of rabbit bone marrow-derived mesenchymal stem cells in polymeric scaffolds. *Biomaterials Research* **7**(2): 120–127.

D

Protocol of Chondrogenesis from BMSC on a Porcine Chondrocytes-Derived Extracellular Matrix Scaffold

Soon Hee Kim*
Kyoung-Hwan Choi†
Byoung-Hyun Min*,†

Background

- Damaged articular cartilage has a limited potential to regenerate due to

*Corresponding Author.
†Cell Therapy Center, Department of Orthopedic Surgery and Department of Molecular Sci & Tech, Ajou University, Suwon 442-721, Korea.

avascularity and the presence of relatively few cells with low mitotic activity. Surgical treatment often induces fibrous repair tissues and unsatisfactory function. In the case of autologous chondrocyte transplantation (ACI), it is hard to harvest many cells from autologous cartilage because of the low cell density of native cartilage tissue. Stem cells have generated significant interest in cartilage tissue engineering as an alternative to autologous chondrocytes because of their ability to differentiate into chondrocytes, ease of isolation and self-renewal. BMSCs have been investigated for chondrogenesis in a variety of culture conditions.

- The microenvironment of biomaterial scaffolds is very important for cellular functions, stem cell differentiation, tissue formation and eventually regeneration of injured tissues. ECM materials have various physiological functions by acting as a reservoir of cytokines and growth factors, transmitting specific signals through interactions with cell surface receptors, and providing specific microenvironments similar to natural tissues.

- Porcine chondrocytes-derived ECM scaffold consists of cartilage matrix molecules mainly including GAGs. This ECM scaffold is biodegradable, biocompatible and highly porous in nature. In addition, this scaffold is efficient at producing high quality hyaline cartilage-like tissues using chondrocytes.

- We introduce the method on chondrogenesis of BMSCs in porcine chondrocytes-derived ECM scaffold. This tissue engineering technique will play a positive role in generating cartilage tissues.

Preparation of ECM Scaffolds[1,2]

- Harvest articular cartilage from 2–3 weeks-old pigs and dissect cartilage pieces.
- Wash with PBS and treat with 0.05% (w/v) pronase at 37°C for 1.5 hr.
- Wash the cartilage pieces twice with PBS and treat 0.2% (w/v) collagenase for 15 hr in DMEM supplemented with 5% NCS.
- Centrifuge the isolated chondrocytes at $600 \times g$ for 10 min.

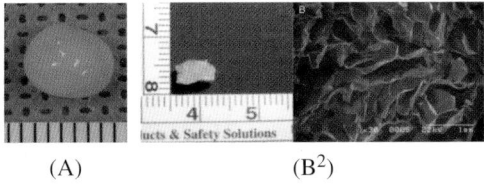

(A)   (B²)

Fig. 1 (A) The gross morphology of consolidated membrane; (B) exterior and inside structure of ECM scaffold. ECM scaffold is a sponge type with uniformly distributed pores and white in color.

- Wash cell pellets with medium twice and seed them in tissue culture plates at a density of 1.9×10^5 cells per plate.
- Culture cells in monolayer with DMEM supplemented with 10% NCS, 1% antibiotic–antimyotics, and 50 µg/mL L-ascorbic acid.
- Remove the medium after 3–4 days and add 0.05% EDTA to separate a chondrocyte/ECM membrane from the bottom of the culture plate.
- Isolate the membrane with a wide-bore pipette and transfer it to a 50-mL conical tube filled with 30 mL DMEM and 5% NCS.
- Centrifuge the tube at $600 \times g$ for 20 min to consolidate the membrane into a pellet type construct and incubate it overnight at 37°C.
- Transfer the construct to a six-well culture plate and culture it for 3 weeks with the culture medium changed 3 times a week.
- After 3 weeks, wash the construct with PBS and then store it at −20°C for 3 days (Fig. 1).
- In order to fabricate an ECM scaffold, freeze-dry the construct for 48 hr at −56°C under 5 mTorr.
- In order to decellularize scaffold, treat with 200 U/mL DNase I and wash with PBS 3 times.
- Trim the construct to 6 mm of diameter and 2–3 mm of thickness (Fig. 1).

Isolation and Culture of rBMSCs[1]

- Aspirate bone marrow aseptically from the tibia and femur of 2-weeks-old female New Zealand white rabbits.

- Obtain mononuclear cells (MNCs) by Ficoll-gradient centrifugation at 1500 × g for 5 min.
- Re-suspend MNCs in α-MEM supplemented with 1% antibiotic-antimycotic and 10% FBS.
- Seed MNCs at 1.5×10^6 cells/plate (150 mm) and culture it at 37°C in a 5% CO_2 incubator.
- After 2 days, remove non-adherent cells and further culture only adherent cells.
- At day 14 after cell seeding, retrieve the adherent rBMSCs by trypsin treatment and replate them at 1×10^6 cells/plate (150 mm) for expansion.

Chondrogenic Differentiation of rBMSCs *In Vitro* and *In Vivo*

- Wash the ECM scaffold 3 times with PBS containing antibiotics and pre-incubate the scaffolds in chondrogenic defined medium (DMEM supplemented with ITS mixture, 50 μg/mL ascorbate 2-phosphate, 100 nM dexamethasone, 40 mg/mL proline, and 1.25 mg/mL BSA) for 12 hr at 37°C.
- Prepare 5×10^6 cells in 1 mL medium and load dynamically into an ECM scaffold for 90 min.
- Place the cell-seeded scaffolds in 24-well plate and incubate until 1 week at 37°C under 5% CO_2 in chondrogenic medium to induce pre-chondrogenic differentiation.
- Implant the cell-seeded scaffolds to back subcutaneous site of six-week-old male nude mice.

Analysis for Chondrogenesis in ECM Scaffold *In Vitro* and *In Vivo*

- Gross observation related with shape, size and color
- Chemical stains: Safranin-O/Fast Green to confirm accumulated sulfated proteoglycan, von Kossa for calcified tissues, Gomori aldehyde fuchsin for elastin fiber, Hematoxylin/Eosin to visualize cell distribution and morphology
- Immunohistochemical analysis for type II collagen, type I collagen, type X collagen, osteocalcin, CD31 and endostatin

- Lacunae observation as evidence of chondrogenesis by histology
- RT-PCR analysis for type II collagen and SOX-9 mRNA.

Requirements

Pronase, collagenase, newborn calf serum, antibiotic–antimyotic, l-ascorbic acid, EDTA, deoxyribonuclease (DNase) I, Ficoll, a-MEM, ITS mixture, ascorbate 2-phosphate, dexamethasone, proline, bovine serum albumin (BSA), DMEM, PBS, FBS.

Characterization

- Extracted samples should be observed in terms of scaffold appearance and chondrogenesis-related protein production and mRNA expression by histology and RT-PCR, respectively. Chondrogenic phenotypes in seeded cells could be decreased over time in scaffolds. The loss of chondrogenic phenotypes appeared to accompany increases in calcification of the matrix and hypertrophic changes. In addition, these hypertrophic changes and calcification of matrix are known to be followed by vessel invasion. Therefore, factors related with calcification, hypertrophic changes and vessel invasion also should be examined with chondrogenic factors.
- Extracted ECM scaffold shows whitish, hyaline cartilage-like morphology. This morphology is similar to native articular cartilage (Fig. 2A).
- The RT-PCR analysis shows that the mRNA of type II collgen and Sox-9 was maintained at high levels at all time points (Fig. 2B).
- Differentiated chondrocytes are characterized by a rounded morphology and the production of ECM molecules such as sulfated GAGs and type II collagen. Red color in Safranin-O/Fast Green staining that indicates accumulation of sulfated GAGs shows at high levels in ECM scaffold (Fig. 3A). The differentiated cells in the metachromatically stained area of the ECM scaffold during the entire implantation period were

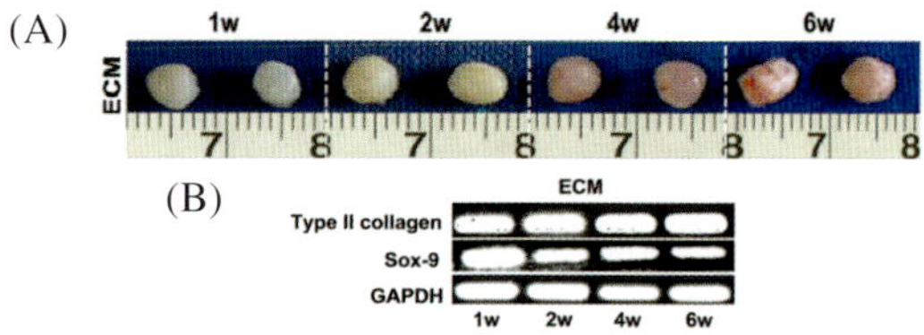

Fig. 2 (A) The gross images of specimens. (B) Expression levels of type II collagen, sox-9 and GAPDH by RT-PCR analysis. The implanted specimens were retrieved at 1, 2, 4 and 6 weeks after implantation.[1]

predominantly rounded in morphology and encapsulated in lacunae structures, which is similar to chondrocytes in native cartilage. Agglomerated chondrocytes were distributed evenly over ECM scaffold. In the immunostaining for type II collagen, a strong expression of type II collagen was in the whole samples (Fig. 3B).

- To examine if the loss of chondrogenic phenotypes was correlated with calcification of the matrix, von Kossa staining was carried out for the samples retrieved from the implantation (Fig. 4). Black stains (indicative of calcified mineral deposits) were observed in the peripheral region and spread into the central region with time. However, the degree of extension was slighter than other synthetic scaffolds (data not shown). This tendency would be correlated oppositely with the positive area of the Safranin-O/Fast Green staining.

- To examine if the loss of chondrogenic phenotypes was correlated with hypertrophy or degeneration of cartilage, immunostaining for type I and type X collagen and osteocalcin was performed (Fig. 4). The expressions of type X collagen, type I collagen and osteocalcin would be found in the same region.

- To examine if the hypertrophic changes and calcification accompany vessel invasion, immunostaining for endostatin, CD31 (PECAM) and Gomori aldehyde fuchsin for elastin fiber was performed (Fig. 4). The expression of endostatin and CD31 was observed only in the peripheral area of the ECM scaffolds, which is similar with the expression patterns of type I and X collagen and osteocalcin.

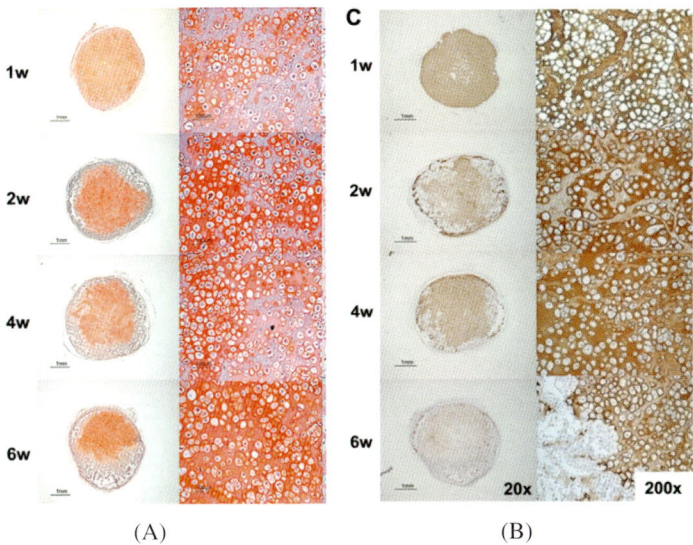

Fig. 3 Histology for chondrogenesis confirmation. The sections were (A) stained Safranin-O/Fast Green (to see accumulation of sulfated proteoglycans), (B) immunostained with an antibody against rabbit type II collagen (to see type II collagen production). The implanted specimens were retrieved at 1, 2, 4 and 6 weeks after implantation. The stained images are presented as a whole sample (first column, magnified ×20) and at high magnification (second columns, ×200). Scale bar 1 mm for ×20 and 100 μm for ×200 images.[1]

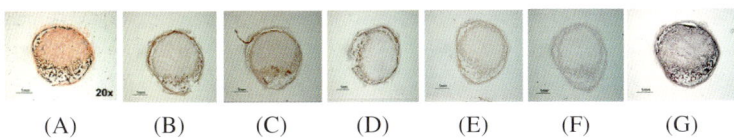

Fig. 4 Histology for calcification, hypertrophic changes and vessel invasion. The sections were (A) stained von Kossa (to see calcium deposit), immunostained with an antibody against (B) type I collagen, (C) type X collagen, (D) osteocalcin to observe calcification and hypertrophic changes. The sections were immunostained with an antibody against (E) endostatin, (F) CD31 and stained with (G) Gomori aldehyde fuchsin to observe vessel invasion. The implanted specimens were retrieved at 1, 2, 4 and 6 weeks after implantation magnified ×20, scale bar; 1 mm magnified ×200, Scale bar; 200 μm).

- Taken together, these results suggest that the ECM scaffold is efficient not only for chondrogenic differentiation but also for the maintenance of chondrogenic phenotypes *in vivo*.

Note

- Submerge ECM scaffolds in 99% alcohol for 10 hr for sterilization and keep at 4°C before use.

References

1. KH Choi, BH Choi, SR Park, *et al.* (2010) The chondrogenic differentiation of mesenchymal stem cells on an extracellular matrix scaffold derived from porcine chondrocytes. *Biomaterials* **31:** 5355–5365.
2. CZ Jin, SR Park, BH Choi, *et al.* (2007) *In vivo* cartilage tissue engineering using a cell-derived extracellular matrix scaffold. *Artificial Organs* **31**(3): 183–192.

E

Protocol of Chondrogenesis of MSC by Ultrasonication

Byoung-Hyun Min*, So Ra Park† and Hyun Jung Lee*

---

* Cell Therapy Center, Ajou University, Suwon, 443-270, Korea.

†Department of Physiology, Inha University College of Medicine, Incheon, 440-712, Korea.

Background

- Ultrasound (US) is a special type of sonic wave with a high frequency above the limit of human audibility of 2–20 kHz. The frequency of US around 3–10 MHz is used in general in clinical applications, mainly for diagnostic and therapeutic purposes. Therapeutic US has diverse intensities and frequencies depending on the purpose of applications, but it can be divided into two main biological functions: thermal and non-thermal effects. Non-thermal effects of US are generally associated with the low intensity ultrasound (LIUS) of less than 1 W/cm².

- LIUS has positive effects on the (i) viability of chondrocytes and MSCs in 3D culture; (ii) chondrocyte proliferation in monolayer culture; (iii) matrix protein synthesis at the transcriptional level; (iv) matrix integrity by regulating the levels of TIMPs and MMPs; (v) chondrogenic differentiation of MSCs *in vitro* and *in vivo*; and (vi) repair of cartilage damage *in vivo*.

Use of Low-Intensity Ultrasound (LIUS) for the Chondrogenic Differentiation of Mesenchymal Stem Cells *In Vitro*

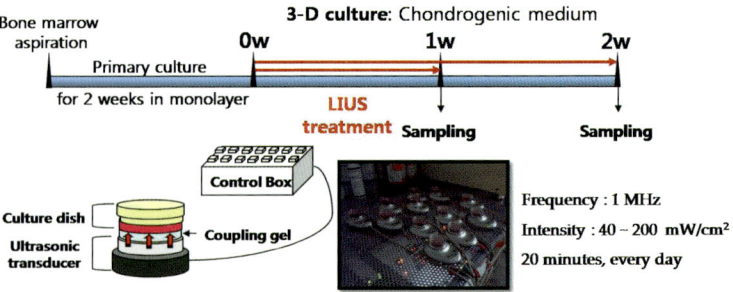

Fig. 1 Diagram showing the experimental schemes for the exposure to LIUS of MSCs grown in alginate culture.[1]

Preparation of MSCs

- MSCs were isolated from bone of animal or human.
- Bone marrow aspirates were obtained aseptically from the tibia and femur by flushing several times with PBS, and marrow was extruded by inserting a 22 gauge needle into the shaft of the bone.
- The bone marrow aspirates from the tibia and femur were suspended in 5% acetic acid and then centrifuged at 1500 rpm for 5 min to remove the red blood cells.
- The cell pellets were re-suspended in MEM supplemented with antibiotics and 10% NCS.
- Cells of 1.5×10^7 were seeded in a tissue culture plate (150 mm dia.) and cultured in monolayer for 2 weeks at 37°C in 5% CO_2 incubator.
- Attached cells (MSCs) were then retrieved using 0.05% trypsin-EDTA followed by centrifugation at 1500 rpm for 10 min.
- Being re-suspended in the same culture medium, cells were plated again at 1.5×10^6 cells per plate and culture expanded with the medium changed three times a week.
- At day 14 from the initial plating, cells were passaged by the trypsin treatment as above (passage 1).
- After 1 week, the cells at passage 2 were used for chondrogenic differentiation in a 3D alginate culture with LIUS treatment.

Three-dimensional (3D) environment for chondrogenic differentiation-alginate culture

- When the secondary culture of MSCs (passage 2) was about 80% confluent, cells were trypsinized and suspended in a 2% alginate solution at a density of 2×10^6 cells/mL.
- The cell/alginate mixture of 200 μL was added slowly in a 12-well transwell insert and spread evenly on the surface.
- The transwell was then immersed in 1 mL of sterile 102 mM $CaCl_2$ solution for 15 min. The MSCs/alginate layer was then washed twice with 0.15 M NaCl for 10 min each and once with serum-free chondrogenic defined medium containing DMEM, ITS supplement (1.0 mg/mL insulin from bovine pancreas, 0.55 mg/mL human transferring and 0.5 μg/mL sodium selenite), 50 μg/mL L-ascorbic acid 2-phosphate, 100 nM

dexamethasone, 40 µg/mL proline, 1.25 mg/mL BSA and 100 µg/mL sodium pyruvate. Alginate layers were then moved to 35 mm culture dishes (7 alginate layers/dish) and overlaid with serum-free chondrogenic defined medium for treatment.

Treatment of LIUS

- The equipment used for ultrasonic stimulation was Ultrasound system (Cell Therapy Center, Ajou University, Suwon, Korea) that has 12 transducers of 35 mm in diameter and controllers to adjust the intensity and time.
- The cell culture dishes were placed directly on the surface of transducers pre-coated with a coupling gel to secure direct contact.
- LIUS stimulation was performed for 20 min every day until the assays at a frequency of 1 MHz and an intensity of 40–200 mW/cm^2 (a condition for cell proliferation in monolayer culture: 100 mW/cm^2) in a continuous wave fashion.
- During the LIUS treatment, the cultures were incubated in a humidified incubator at 37°C under 5% CO_2 for 1 or 2 weeks with the culture medium changed every other day.

Use of Low-Intensity Ultrasound (LIUS) for the Chondrogenic Differentiation of Mesenchymal Stem Cells *In Vivo*

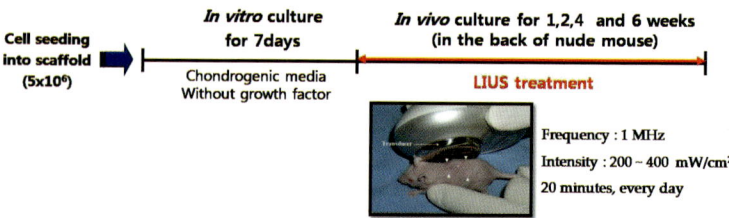

Fig. 2 A diagram showing an experimental scheme for the exposure to LIUS of PGA/MSC constructs grown in the back of nude mice *in vivo*. A coupling gel was used for efficient US delivery between transducer and target areas in the back of nude mouse. The markings in arrow shape indicate the implantation sites of the PGA/MSC constructs.[2]

Isolation and culture of rabbit MSCs

- MSCs were isolated from two-week-old female New Zealand white rabbits (Joong-Ang Experimental Animal Center, Seoul, Korea).
- The bone marrow aspirates from the tibia and femur were suspended in 5% acetic acid and then centrifuged at 1500 rpm for 5 min to remove red blood cells (RBCs).
- The cell pellets were re-suspended in MEM supplemented with antibiotics and 10% NCS.
- Cells of 1.5×10^7 were seeded in tissue culture plate (150 mm dia.) and cultured in monolayer for 2 weeks at 37°C in 5% CO_2 incubator.
- Attached cells were then retrieved using 0.05% trypsin-EDTA followed by centrifugation at 1500 rpm for 10 min.
- Being re-suspended in the same culture medium, cells were plated again at 1.5×10^6 cells per plate and culture expanded with the medium changed three times a week. The second passaged cells were used for seeding into the PGA scaffold.

Preparation of PGA/MSCs constructs

- Biodegradable PGA non-woven mesh (Albany International. INC, Mansfield, MA) was used as a scaffold for 3D MSCs culture. The PGA mesh was cut into pieces to have an equal dimension (5 mm × 5 mm × 3 mm).
- They were submerged in 70% alcohol for 10 hr to be sterilized and kept at 4°C before MSCs seeding.
- Washed three times with antibiotics-included PBS, the PGA scaffolds were held in DMEM and stayed for 12 hr at 37°C incubator.
- The passaged MSCs were then statically seeded at 5×10^6 cells per scaffold.
- The culture medium was a chondrogenic-defined medium, DMEM supplemented with ITS, 50 µg/mL L-ascorbic acid 2-phosphate, 100 nM dexamethasone, 40 mg/mL proline, 1.25 mg/mL BSA, and 10% NCS. They were cultured for a week before nude mouse implantation.

In vivo Implantation and LIUS Stimulation

- Five-week-old male nude mice (n = 9, each group) were anesthetized with a mixture of ketamine hydrochloride and rumpun.
- The back skin of nude mouse was incised for the implantation of MSC-seeded PGA scaffold into the subcutaneous tissue. Total of four specimens were implanted at a time per mouse. Two were placed longitudinally at one side of the back and another two were positioned at the other side.
- On the following day, LIUS stimulation was given to one side first for 10 min and switched to the other side for another 10 min.
- An ultrasound device (Cell Therapy Center, Ajou University, Suwon, Korea) was used for the stimulation that was applied every day for 1, 2 and 4 weeks, respectively, at a frequency of 1 MHz and intensity of 200–400 mW/cm^2 in a continuous wave mode.
- Control mice were prepared in the same manner and grown without the exposure to LIUS.

Analysis for Chondrogenesis by Ultrasonication

Effects of LIUS on the viability of MSCs

- Live/Dead Viability/Cytotoxicity assay (Molecular Probe, Eugene, OR).

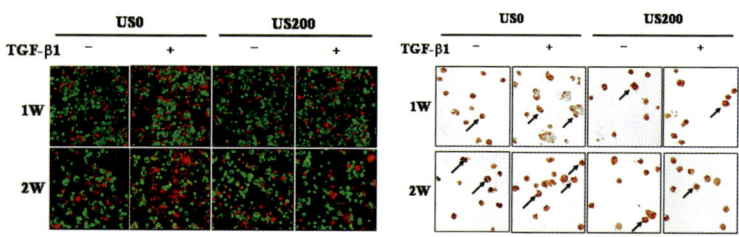

Fig. 3 Effects of LIUS on the hMSCs viability and apoptosis by live/dead viability/cytotoxicity assay and FragEL DNA fragmentation detection assay.[2]

- Apoptosis analysis using a Colorimetric FragEL DNA fragmentation Detection Kit (Calbiochem, San Diego, CA).
- RT-PCR for bax and bcl-2 expression.

Effects of LIUS on the proliferation of MSCs

- $_3$H-thymidine incorporation.
- Trypan blue exclusion method.
- MTT assay.

Effects of LIUS on the ECM synthesis of MSCs

- $_{35}$S-sulfate incorporation for proteoglycan synthesis rate.
- $_3$H-proline uptake for collagen synthesis.
- Histological analysis (Safranin-O or Alcian Blue staining) for proteoglycan and immunohistochemical (type I and type II collagen) evaluation.
- DMMB assay for sulfated GAG contents.

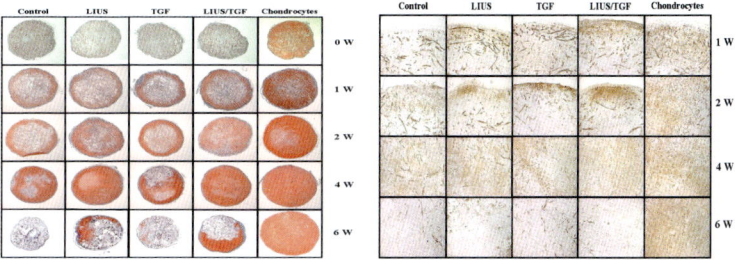

Fig. 4 Histologic features of Safranin-O/Fast Green staining and immunohistochemistry of type II collagen for the implanted constructs at different time points.[2]

References

1. HJ Lee, BH Choi, BH Min, SR Park. (2007) Low-intensity ultra sound inhibits apoptosis and enhances viability of human mesen-chymal stem cells in three-dimensional alginate culture during chondrogenic differentiation. *Tissue Eng* **13**(5): 1049–1057.
2. JH Cui, SR Park, K Park, *et al.* (2007) Preconditioning of mesen-chymal stem cell with low-intensity ultrasound for cartilage for-mation *in vivo*. *Tissue Eng* **13**(2): 351–360.

F

Protocol of Chondrogenesis of BMSC to Chondrocyte Using Chitosan-Modified Poly(L-Lactide-*co*-ε-Caprolactone) Scaffolds

Zheng Yang[,§], Xiaoyan Tang[†], Chao Li[†] and Zigang Ge[†,‡,§]*

[*]NUS Tissue Engineering Program, Life Sciences Institute, National University of Singapore, 27 Medical Dr, Singapore 117510.

[†]Department of Biomedical Engineering, College of Engineering and [‡]Center for Biomedical materials and Tissue Engineering, Academy for Advanced Interdisciplinary Studies, Peking University, Beijing 100871, China. [§]Center for Joint Diseases, Peking University Renmin Hospital, Beijing, P. R. China

Background

- Articular cartilage is an avascular connective tissue distinct from most tissues that has only limited self-regeneration ability. Chondral lesions are unable to self-repair spontaneously due to the lack of migration of the resident chondrocytes and the progenitor cells from the blood or the bone marrow as a result of the absence of vasculature.[1,2]

- Among the more successful approaches, cell-based approaches using both autologous chondrocyte implantations (ACI) and autologous MSC implantation have both led to symptomatic improvement clinically.[3,4]

- Successful cartilage tissue engineering using stem cells will require the delivery of the cells in carrier scaffolds that provide suitable biomechanical and biocompatible properties to the implanted tissue. As articular cartilage is a weight-bearing tissue with viscoelastic properties that endow cartilage with the unique capability to withstand continuous complex mechanical loading, the scaffold should exhibit appropriate elastomeric properties.

- In this chapter, we present the protocols for the chondrogenic differentiation of MSCs in an elastomeric chitosan-modified poly(L-lactide-co-ε-caprolactone) (PLCL) scaffold,[5,6] and the immunohistochemical and RNA analytical methods for confirmation of cartilage tissue formation.

Fabrication of PLCL Scaffold and Cross-Linking of Chitosan

Fabrication of PLCL scaffold

- Dissolve PLCL (7:3) in 1,4-dioxane (10% w/v) and mix with a proportional amount of sodium chloride (NaCl).[5]

- After agitation, cast the NaCl/PLCL mixtures in glass molds and then freeze at −20°C for 24 hr.

- Immerse the frozen mixtures in a 70% ethanol aqueous solution that was pre-cooled to −20°C for 72 hr.

- After substituting the solvent and part of the NaCl with ethanol aqueous solution, lyophilize the mixtures in a freeze dryer for 24 hr to form the desired PLCL scaffold.

Aminolysis of PLCL scaffold and chitosan immobilization

- Immerse scaffolds in a 50% ethanol solution for 2 hr to remove any oil on the scaffold surface before reacting in a 10% (w/v) 1,6-hexanediamine/isopropanol solution at 37°C for 10 min.
- Immerse scaffolds into a 1% glutaraldehyde solution at room temperature for 3 hr before rinsing with distilled water.
- Incubate scaffolds in 2 mg/mL chitosan solution (pH = 3.5) at 2–4°C for 24 hr, then rinse with 0.1 N acetic acid solution before rinsing with distilled water.
- Place acquired dried scaffolds (Fig. 1) in the vacuum chamber and store in a dessicator until further usage.

Isolation and Culture of BMSC

- Isolate human bone marrow mononuclear cells from the iliac crest bone marrow aspirate by using RosetteSep® Human

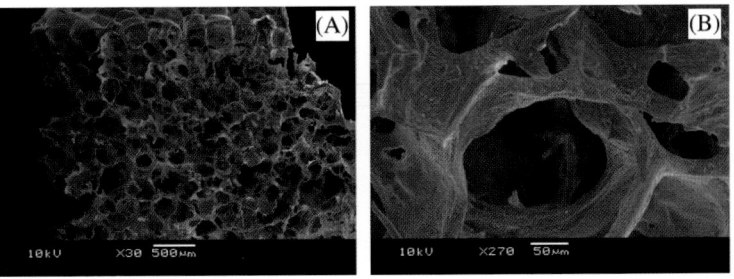

Fig. 1 SEM images of a chitosan-modified PLCL scaffold at two magnifications (A: ×30 and B: ×270 magnification).

Mesenchymal Stem Cell Enrichment Cocktail (Note 1). Re-suspend the isolated mononuclear cells in MSC expansion media (DMEM supplemented with 10% FBS (Note 2) and 100U/100µg P/S), seed cells in T75 tissue culture flask and incubate in 37°C incubator. Non-adherent cells are removed 4–5 days after plating, and adherent MSC allowed to proliferate in expansion media until they reach 90% confluence. Replace the medium every 3–4 days.

- To further expand the MSC, the media is aspirated, followed by enzymatic-treatment with 2 mL of 0.25% trypsin/EDTA at 37°C for 5 min. The tissue culture flask is lightly tapped on the side to help lift off the cells. Treatment is inactivated with addition of 8 mL of expansion media. Cells are counted and seeded at 4×10^3 cells per cm^2.

Chondrogenic Differentiation of MSC

Chondrogenic differentiation of MSC is carried out in the chitosan/PLCL system.[6]

- Prepare chondrogenic medium by mixing the following in a 50 mL screw cap tube: 47 mL DMEM high-glucose, 5 µL of 10 mM Dexamethasone and 0.5 mL of each of the following stock solutions: GlutaMax-I Supplement, penicillin/streptomycin, sodium pyruvate, ITS^{+1}, 5 mg/mL ascorbic acid 2-phosphate, 0.4 M L-proline. Chondrogenic medium can be kept for up to 1 month at 4°C. Warm to 37°C in a water bath before use. Add TGF-β3 to the chondrogenic medium at 1 µL of TGF-β3 stock solution (long/µL) to each 1 mL of the cell suspension, giving the final TGF-β3 concentration of 10 ng/mL.
- Harvest MSC by trypsinisation. Ensure cells are less than 90% confluent at the time of harvest. Collect cells by centrifugation at $200 \times g$ for 5 min. Re-suspend cells in MSC expansion media. Count the cells and adjust the volume of the suspension to 10×10^6 cells per mL.
- Cut PLCL/chitosan scaffold into $4 \times 4 \times 2$ mm size. Sterilize the scaffold with 70% ethanol for 1 hr, immerse scaffold 3×10 min with PBS to remove ethanol then immerse it in PBS until use.

- Before cell seeding, blot the scaffold dry with sterilized filter paper and place it in the well of 24-well plate. Immediately seed 25 µL of MSC at 10×10^6 cells per mL onto the scaffold, letting the cell suspension to soak into the scaffold by gravitation force.

- Incubate the cell/scaffold in 37°C incubator for 2 hr to allow cell adhesion to the scaffold, before slowing adding 1 mL of MSC expansion media into the well. Incubate the samples in 37°C incubator overnight.

- Chondrogenic differentiation is started by replacing the expansion media with 1 mL of chondrogenic differentiation media. Replace the medium every 2–3 days with fresh chondrogenic medium.

Analysis of Chondrogenic Matrix Protein Synthesis

Preparation of chondrogenic tissue sections for histology and immunohistochemistry

- After completion of chondrogenesis, the medium is removed from the samples.

- Immerse the samples in embedding medium Tissue-Tek O.C.T compound and freeze down at −20°C.

- Cut 10 µm sections using a cryosection microtome and transfer them to Superfrost®Plus microscope slides. The cut tissue section at room temperature for 30 min to facilitate adherence of the section to the slide. Tissues on the sections are fixed in ice cold fixative solution (acetone/methanol 1:1 v/v) for 15 min. Slides are again air dry for 30 min and store in 4°C before use.

- Immediately before staining, the tissues are rehydrated in PBS.

Histological staining for proteoglycan (Alcian Blue and Nuclear Fast Red staining)

- Stain the rehydrated sections on microscope slides with 0.5% Alcian Blue solution (pH = 2.5) for 30 min. Then rinse in distilled water 3×3 min.

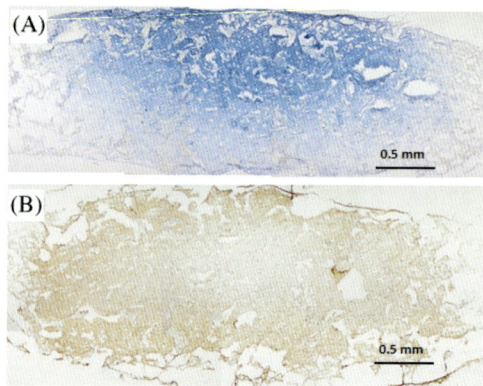

Fig. 2 MSC was differentiated into chondrogenic lineage for 21 days in the presence of TGF-β3. Proteoglycan deposition was analyzed by Alcian Blue (A), and type II collagen was analyzed by immunohisto-chemical staining (B).

- Stain the nuclei of the cells with nuclear Nuclear Fast Red for 5 minutes, then rinse slides briefly in two changes of 95% ethanol followed by two changes of 100% ethanol.
- Wash in xylene, air-dry and coverslip.
- An example of the Alcian Blue-stained chondrogenic section of PLCL/chitosan scaffold construct is shown in Fig. 2A.

Immunostaining for collagen proteins

Collagen type II expression is detected by immunohistochemis-try using the UltraVision HRP Detection System.

- Using a wax pen, draw a circle on the microscope slide to surround the rehydrated sections. Add a drop of hydrogen peroxide block to the tissue section within the wax circle and incubate for 15 min. Wash 2 × 5 min with PBS.
- Incubate tissue sections under drops of pepsin at 37°C for 15 min and then wash 2 × 5 min with PBS.
- Incubate in Ultra V Block for 5 min (Note 3).

- Drain excess Ultra V Block (Note 4) and then add 0.2 mg/mL of the type II collagen primary antibody or matching isotype control (mouse IgG1). After incubation at room temperature for 1 hr, wash the sections 4 × 2 min in PBS.
- Incubate the sections with biotinylated goat anti-mouse for 30 min then wash the sections 4 × 2 min in PBS.
- Incubate the sections with strepavidin peroxidase for 45 min then wash 4 × 2 min in PBS.
- Prepare color development substrate by mixing 1 drop DAB chromagen with 1 mL of DAB substrate and mix by inverting tube.
- Add the color development substrate to the sections and incubate until staining is evident (1–3 min). Remove the color solution and stop the reaction by immersing the slides in distilled water.
- Counterstain the sections with hematoxylin.
- Example of the collagen-stained chondrogenic section of PLCL/chitosan scaffold construct is shown in Fig. 2B.

Analysis of Cartilage-Specific Genes

Total RNA extraction and cDNA synthesis

- Remove the differentiation medium from the sample and digest the extracellular matrix with 1 mL of 0.25% collagenase for 1 hr at 37°C water bath to release the cells. Centrifuge at 200 × g to pellet the cells. Remove the medium and extract total RNA from the cells using the RNeasy Mini Kit (Qiagen), following the manufacturer's instructions.
- Determine the RNA quantity and quality by measuring the absorbance at 260 nm and 280 nm for each samples using the Nanodrop ND-1000 spectrophotometer. Calculate the RNA concentration of the sample: 1 unit at 260 nm corresponds to 40 µg of RNA per mL. A260/A280 ratio of 1.8–2.0 indicates good purity of the extracted RNA. Store the RNA samples at −80°C if cDNA synthesis is not carried out on the day itself.
- Place reverse transcriptase reaction in a PCR thermal cycler. Perform cDNA synthesis by using 50–100 ng of total RNA

per 20 µL reaction volume over a 30 min incubation time at 42°C, with the addition of 5 × iScript Biorad reaction mix and 1 µL iScript reverse transcriptase, followed by enzyme inactivation at 85°C for 5 min, according to the manufacturer's instructions.

Quantitative real-time polymerase chain reaction (RT-PCR)

- Analyze Sox9, Aggrecan and Col 2 gene expression by real-time RT-PCR reactions using the SYBR® Green PCR Master Mix System on Real-Time PCR thermocycler (7500 Real Time PCR System; Applied Biosystems).
- cDNA samples (1 µL for a total volume of 20 µL per reaction) were analyzed for gene of interest normalized to reference gene glyceraldehydes-3-phosphate dehydrogenase (*GAPDH*). The level of expression of each target gene is then calculated as $2^{-\Delta\Delta Ct}$, with reference to the undifferentiated MSC.
- RT-PCR is performed at 95°C for 10 min followed by 40 cycles of 15 sec denaturation at 95°C, and an extension step at 60°C for 1 min. PCR primers are listed in Table 1.
- Example of Sox9, Aggrecan and Col2 gene expression levels of human MSC differentiation in PLCL/chitosan scaffold is shown in Fig. 3.

Table 1   RT-PCR primers

Gene	Primer sequence
Sox9	Forward: 5′-CAGTACCCGCACTTGCACAA-3′ Reverse: 5′-CTCGTTCAGAAGTCTCCAGAGCTT-3′
Aggrecan	Forward: 5′-ACTTCCGCTGGTCAGATGGA-3′ Reverse: 5′-TCTCGTGCCAGATCATCACC-3′
Col2	Forward: 5′-GGCAATAGCAGGTTCACGTACA-3′ Reverse: 5′-CGATAACAGTCTTGCCCCACTT-3′
GAPDH	Forward: 5′-ATGGGGAAGGTGAAGGTCG-3′ Reverse: 5′-TAAAAGCAGCCCTGGTGACC-3′

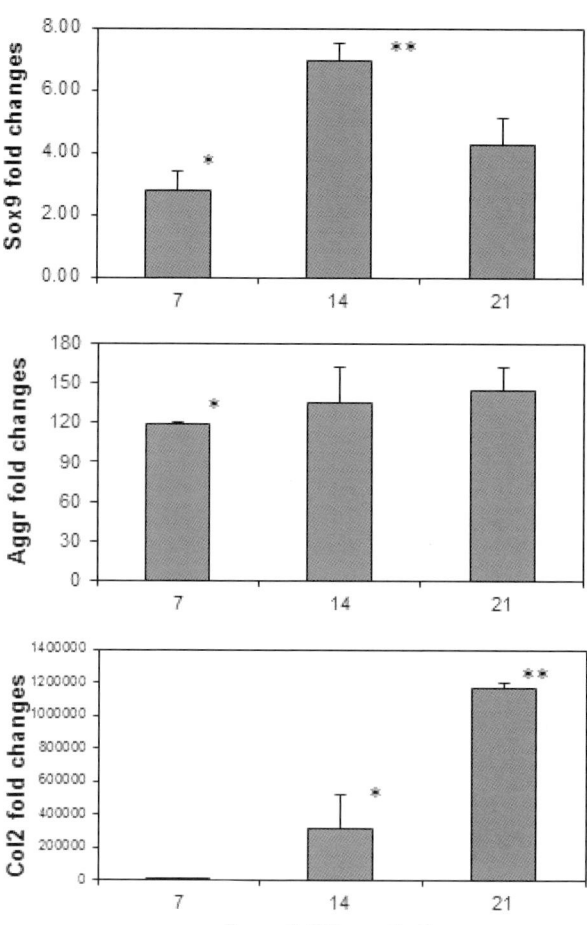

Fig. 3 Real-time PCR quantification of chondrogenic marker Sox9, aggrecan (Aggr) and type II collagen (Col2) in PLCL/chitosan constructs. Expression was normalized to GAPDH and presented as fold changes relative to level in undifferentiated MSC. Data shown are means ± SD (n = 5). *p < 0.05 significant increase in PLCL/chitosan construct undifferentiated MSC. **p < 0.05 significant increase between time points.

Notes

1. Isolation of mononuclear cells from bone marrow aspirate using RosetteSep® Human Mesenchymal Stem Cell Enrichment Cocktail follows exactly the recommendation of the manufacturer's protocol. (http://www.stemcell.com/technical/15128_15168-PIS.pdf).

2. Source of FBS affects MSC due to variation of yet to be identified components in the serum. To maintain good performance of the expanded MSC, i.e. high proliferation rate and multilineage differentiation capacity, it is recommended that FBS be tested for their ability to support the expansion and clonal enumeration (colony forming unit fibroblast assay) of MSCs, or that commercially available MSC-grade FBS be used.

3. Incubations > 10 min may reduce signal.

4. Do not rinse off the Ultra V Block.

References

1. JA Buckwalter. (1998) Articular cartilage: Injuries and potential for healing. *J Orthop Sports Phys Ther* **28**(4): 192–202.

2. TA Ahmed, MT Hincke. (2010) Strategies for articular cartilage lesion repair and functional restoration. *Tissue Eng Part B Rev* **16**(3): 305–329.

3. S Wakitani, K Imoto, T Yamamoto, *et al.* (2002) Human autologous culture expanded bone marrow mesenchymal cell transplantation for repair of cartilage defects in osteoarthritic knees. *Osteoarthritis Cartilage* **10**(3): 199–206.

4. H Nejadnik, JHP Hui, PF Choong, *et al.* (2010) Autologous bone marrow derived mesenchymal stem cell versus autologous chondrocyte implantation: An observational cohort study. *Am J Sports Med* **38**(6): 1110–1116.

5. C Li, L Wang, Z Yang, *et al.* (2012) A viscoelastic chitosan-modified three-dimensional porous poly(L-lactide-*co*-ε-caprolactone) scaffold for cartilage tissue engineering. *J Biomater Sci, Polymer Ed* **23**: 405–424.

6. Z Yang, Y Wu, C Li, *et al.* (2012) *Tissue Eng Part A* **8**(3–4): 242–251.

G

Protocol of Osteogenesis of BMSCs Using Hydroxyapatite/ Tricalciumphosphate Scaffold

EunAh Lee*, Pamela Gehron Robey† and Youngsook Son*,‡

---

*Musculoskeletal Bioorgan Center, College of Life Sci and Graduate School of Biotech, Kyung Hee Univ, Yongin, Gyeonggi-do, 446-701, Korea.

†Craniofacial and Skeletal Diseases Branch, National Institute of Dental and Craniofacial Disease, NIH, DHHS, Bethesda, Maryland, 20892, USA.

Background

- Bone provides mechanical strength to the body and plays an essential role in movement. In the case of critical-sized bone defects, the healing is not complete. To fill large defects, bone fragments from non-load-bearing sites are transplanted into the defect site.
- However, this is not an ideal approach because donor bone fragments may not be of sufficient quantity or of appropriate shape to fit into the defect site in many cases, and the harvest can cause donor site morbidity.
- Current research progress in tissue engineering approaches for bone regeneration using skeletal stem cells and appropriate bone substitutes shows promise in overcoming these difficulties.
- BMSCs, of which multipotent skeletal stem cells are a subset, are considered the gold standard among different cell sources for bone regeneration. BMSCs form ossicles when subcutaneously transplanted into nude mice. They form not only ectopic bone, but also recreate the bone marrow organ system (BMOS) that contains the hematopoietic stem cell niche.
- When BMSCs are subcutaneously transplanted with an appropriate carrier such as hydroxyapatite (HAp)/tricalcium phosphate (TCP), ectopic bone is formed at the site of transplant. However, some bone substitutes are not good enough for ectopic bone formation, and cannot produce ossicles when they transplanted with BMSCs because they are not osteoconductive. Consequently, the choice of a proper bone substitute is very important because a properly mineralized bone matrix is essential for bone tissue regeneration.
- There are growth factors such as BMP-2 that can induce osteogenesis. However, it was reported that those growth factors abrogate the potential of BMSCs to form BMOS while promoting bone formation. Because the BMSC population contains skeletal stem cells that can make bone matrix on the surface of appropriate bone substitute *in vivo* situation, the osteogenic potential of newly constructed biomaterials should be tested by subcutaneous transplantation without using osteogenic growth factors.

Culture of BMSCs

- Requirements: Standard media consisting of alpha-MEM, 2 mM L-glutamine, 100 U/mL penicillin, 100 µg/mL strepto-mycin sulfate, 10^{-8} M dexamethasone, 10^{-4} M L-ascorbic acid, and 20% of lot-selected FBS.
- Remove any muscle or other soft tissues from the bone.
- Place cleaned bone on petri dish and wash with standard medium.
- Mince bone into pieces and place the medium into tube on ice.
- Add new medium and mince further.
- Place medium into the tube on ice.
- Transfer bone pieces and medium to a new tube and shake vigorously.
- Take the medium and pour through a cell strainer (70 µm mesh) into a new tube to remove cell aggregates.
- To count mononuclear cells, take a small volume and dilute in 3% acetic acid at a 1:100 ratio to make RBC ruptured, which makes easier to count mononuclear cells. The cells in 3% acetic acid cannot be used for the culture.
- Plate the cell suspension at a density of 1×10^6 cells/cm^2.
- Change the medium the next day.
- **Note 1:** When using small animals such as mice or rats, take long bones cleaned of muscles with the epiphyses removed. The bone marrow is flushed from the diaphysis using a 6 mL syringe and #23 needle. The rest of the steps are the same.
- **Note 2:** Reliable results of experiments are obtained with cells within 5th passages. Beyond the 5th passage, the mor-phology of the cells is changed and differentiation capacity is altered.

Test of *In Vitro* Osteogenic Differentiation Potential

- Requirements: Osteogenic media consists of standard media plus 10 nmol/L dexamethasone, 10 mmol/L beta-glycer-phosphate, 50 µg/mL ascorbate phosphate, and 10 nmol/L 1,25 dihydroxyvitamin D$_3$. 2% Alizarin Red S solution.

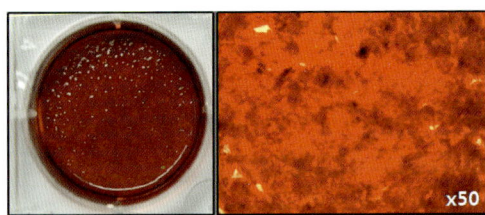

Fig. 1 Test of *in vitro* osteogenic potential of rabbit BMSCs by Alizarin Red staining.

- Cells are suspended in osteogenic media and seeded into 6-well plates at a density of 1×10^4 cells/well.
- Change medium every other day and maintain cultures for 2–3 weeks.
- Determine *in vitro* osteogenic differentiation potential by detection of calcium accumulation using 2% Alizarin Red S staining solution (Fig. 1).

Choice of Bone Substitutes to Test for *In Vivo* Osteogenic Potential

- HAp/TCP (in 60:40 ratio) particle in size range of 0.5–1 mm shows excellent bone formation by subcutaneous transplantation.
- There are some bone substitute particles that are not able to form bone (e.g. poly(lactic acid), poly(glycolic acid) polymers and their derivatives) as shown in Fig. 2.

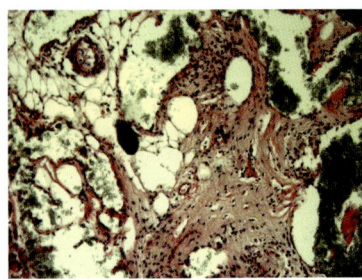
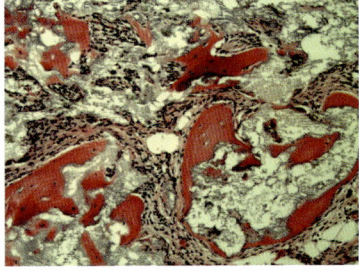

Poor osteogenic scaffold   Highly ostegenic scaffold

Fig. 2 Bone substitutes influence bone formation of BMSCs *in vivo*.

Test of *In Vivo* Osteogenic Differentiation Potential

- Requirement: HAp/TCP (particle sized 0.5–1mm), sterilized by baking.
- Weigh an aliquot of 40 mg of HAp/TCP into a sterile cryovial.
- Wash the HAp/TCP in each vial with medium.
- Put $2–3 \times 10^6$ BMSCs into each vial containing HAp/TCP.
- Put the tubes in a 37°C CO_2 incubator with gentle rotation for 1 hr for the cells to attach to the surface of HAp/TCP.
- Briefly centrifuge and aspirate the media.
- Transplant cells and HAp/TCP mixture subcutaneously into nude mice.
- Sacrifice the mice after 8 weeks and take transplants.
- Proceed for histological analysis.

Tetracycline Labeling to Analyze New Bone Formation

- Requirements: tetracycline in PBS or saline.
- Inject tetracycline at a dose of 200 mg/kg I.P. 3 days before sacrificing the mice bearing transplants.

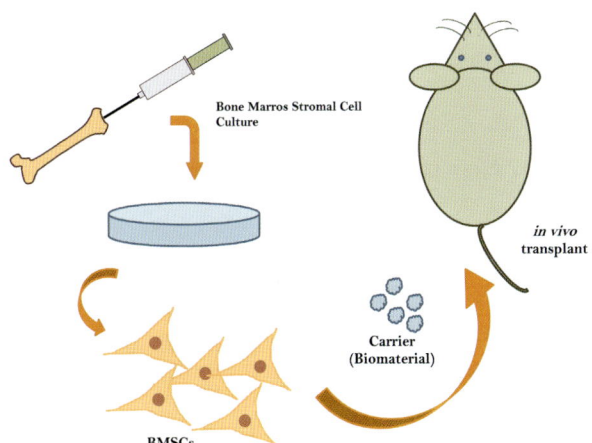

Fig. 3 Test for *in vivo* osteogenic potential by subcutaneous transplant.

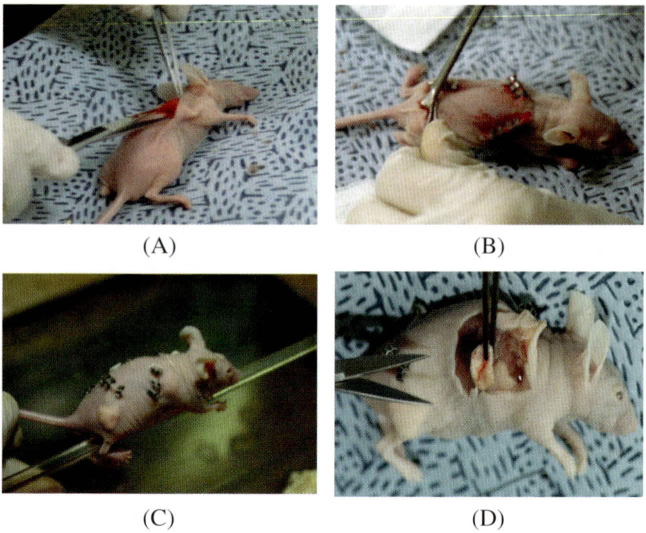

(A) (B)

(C) (D)

Fig. 4 Surgery of subcutaneous transplant. (A) Making an incision on dorsal skin. (B) Transplanting the mixtures of cells and scaffold. (C) Ectopic bones can be seen at the site of transplants. (D) Harvest of transplant.

- Harvest the transplants and embed non-decalcified in methacrylate or cryo-embedding gel for sectioning.
- Check the section under fluorescence microscope.
- Newly formed bone is labeled with tetracycline and visualized as bright yellow fluorescence by UV illumination.

Frozen Sectioning of Bone Samples

- Requirements: cryo-embedding gel, mold for cryo-embedding, cryo-microtome.
- Usually, mineralized hard tissues such as bone should be decalcified to ease the sectioning process. However, it can be sectioned without decalcification using frozen sectioning.
- Place the fixed tissues in cryo-embedding gel in mold, and place the mold on dry ice until hardened.
- Section using a cryo-microtome.
- Keep the sectioned slide frozen until use.

Decalcification for Paraffin Embedding and Sectioning

- Wash the fixed bone tissues with PBS and decalcify in 10% EDTA solution for 2 weeks, or until tissue is demineralized (can be assessed by taking X-rays).
- Change 10% EDTA solution several times during decalcification.
- Wash with tap water before processing for paraffin embedding.
- Subsequent steps for paraffin embedding and sectioning are the same as for soft tissue.

Expected Results of Staining for Bone Sections

- Hematoxylin and Eosin staining: bone matrix (dark solid pink), cytoplasm (pink), nucleus (purple).
- Von Kossa staining: calcified matrix (black).
- Goldner's trichrome staining: nuclei (brownish black), cytoplasm (red), collagen (green).

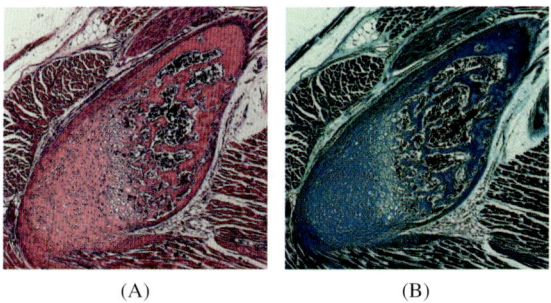

(A)   (B)

Fig. 5 H&E stained (A) and trichrome stained (B) mouse bone sections.

H

Protocol of Osteogenesis from BMSC Cultured with Dexamethasone-Loaded Dendrimer Nanoparticles onto Ceramic and Polymeric Scaffolds: *In Vivo* Studies

Joaquim Miguel Oliveira[*,†,§],
João F. Mano[*,†]*, Hajime
Ohgushi*[‡]*, and Rui Luís Reis*[*,†]

*3B's Research Group — Biomaterials,
Biodegradables and Biomimetics, University of
Minho, Headquarters of the European Institute
of Excellence on Tissue Engineering and
Regenerative Medicine, AvePark, S. Cláudio de
Barco, Caldas das Taipas, Guimarães, Portugal.

Background

- MSCs are a valuable therapeutic tool as they can differentiate either *in vitro* or *in vivo* into osteoblasts under the effect of osteogenic factors such as dexamethasone (Dex).
- The use of dendrimer-based nanocarriers[1,2] that are easily internalized by cells is advantageous due to: (i) improving the drugs' solubility, (ii) delivery to the targets where drugs are required, (iii) improved bioavailability, (iv) allowing modulation of the cellular functions in a more effective manner *ex vivo*, and (v) maintaining the cellular phenotype *in vivo* upon re-implantation.
- Scaffolds such as the macroporous hydroxyapatite (HAp) and starch-polycaprolactone (SPCL) possess an adequate architecture for bone tissue engineering applications.
- We propose the combination of stem cells, nanoparticles systems for the intracellular delivery of Dex and either ceramic or polymeric scaffolds as a way to enhance the osteogenic differentiation of rat BMSCs, *in vitro* and *in vivo*.

Isolation and Culturing Methods of rBMSCs from Fischer 344 Syngeneic Rats

Isolation and culturing

- Donor animals should be 7-weeks-old male Fisher 344(F344/N) rats.
- Bone marrow harvesting and cell culture should be carried out in aseptic conditions and the animals sacrificed using an excess of a general anesthetic.
- Right and left femora should be excised by means of using a sterile scalpel or scissors, followed by cleaning soft tissue around femora.
- Femora should be washed several times with sterile PBS solution, pH 7.4, and then the epiphyseal regions of femora removed with help of scissors.

---

† ICVS/3B's — PT Government Associate Laboratory, Braga/Guimarães, Portugal.

‡ Health Research Institute, National Institute of Advanced Industrial Science and Technology (AIST), Osaka, Japan.

- Using a syringe, flush out marrow plug in the femoral shaft with about 15 mL of culture medium (EMEM containing 10% FBS +100 U/mL Penicillin supplemented with 0.1 mg/mL Streptomycin +0.25 ng/mL Amphotericin B) into a 50 mL polystyrene tube.
- Homogenize with a pipette and transfer the medium with marrow into a T75 cm^2 tissue culture polystyrene culture flask/dish containing 15 mL of the culture medium and incubate at 37°C in a humidified atmosphere containing 5% of CO_2.
- Change the culture medium to remove non-adherent cells within a 3-day period followed by changing the medium every 2 days until reaching about 90% confluence.
- The rBMSCs (passage 1, P1) should be release from substratum with 1 mL of 0.05% trypsin-0.53 mM EDTA and centrifuged at 900 rpm for 5 min, and a cell suspension must be prepared and cell number determined using a standard method.

De-Aeration of the HAp and SPCL Scaffolds

- Sterile HAp and SPCL scaffolds should be pre-treated (de-aeration procedure) to prevent air bubble formation in the pores, which can inhibit cell adhesion.
- Place the scaffolds (5 mm diameter and 4 mm height, n = 5) in 10 mL polystyrene tubes with ventilation caps and add 10 mL of culture medium to the scaffolds and close the tubes with the respective caps.
- De-air the scaffolds under vacuum using a 20 mL syringe with an attached 21G needle and then transfer each scaffold into the respective well of a non-adherent 96-well TCPS plate.

In Vivo Osteogenic Differentiation of rBMSCs Seeded onto the Surface of the SPCL Scaffolds and Cultured with Dex-Loaded CMCht/PAMAM Dendrimer Nanoparticles

Preparation of RBMSCs/scaffold constructs

- Donor and recipient animals should be 7-week-old male Fisher 344 (F344/N) rats.

Note: Sub-strains of the Fisher rats should be matched for both donor/recipient.

- *In vitro* expansion of rBMSCs in different culture media, namely: (i) MEM, (ii) MEM supplemented with Dex, and (iii) MEM supplemented with the Dex-loaded CMCht/PAMAM dendrimer nanoparticles.
- Seed the rBMSCs at different cell number (1×10^6 and 2×10^5) onto the surface of each SPCL scaffold.
- Culture cell/scaffolds constructs in MEM complete medium for cell adhesion, overnight.
- Wash the cell/scaffolds constructs with 1 mL of sterile PBS solution, and then constructs are ready for the subcutaneous implantation.

Implantation procedure

- Seven-weeks-old male F344/N rats (syngeneic), same as donor sub-strain and age, must be anesthetized by intraperitoneal injection of pentobarbital at a final concentration of 3.5 mg per 100 g of body weight.
- Wash the skin with tap water followed by 70% ethanol solution, and then stabilization of the rats should be performed in a prone position.
- Administrate a general anesthesia to the rat and then cut the hair at the implantation area.
- In each rat, three or four skin incisions (each 1 cm length) on the dorsal midline below the ear should be made (Fig. 1).
- Each rBMSCs/scaffold construct should be implanted subcutaneously (1.5 cm to 2 cm away from the midline at both right and left sides) into the respective pocket and skin sutured.
- SPCL implants without rBMSCs are used (negative control).
- All animals should receive their usual dietary regimen and no prophylactic medication should be provided post-surgery.
- After 4, 8 or 12 weeks implantation, the animals are sacrificed with an overdose of general anesthetic and the implants retrieved.
- Experiments should be carried out 3 times using a minimum of 3 implants per condition.

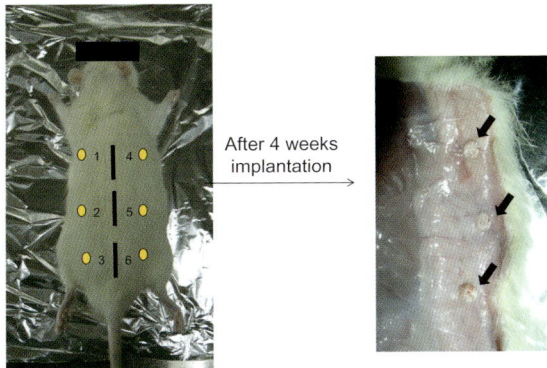

Fig. 1 Subcutaneous implantation sites on the back of F344/N rat. Black arrows indicate the implanted SPCL scaffolds.

Analysis for Osteogenesis *In Vivo*

Micro-CT and morphometric analysis

New bone formation in the polymeric scaffolds is easily evaluated by means of high-resolution micro-computed tomography analysis (e.g. Skyscan 1072 scanner Skyscan, Kontich, Belgium). No processing of the samples is required prior analysis.

Note: The morphometric analysis can include explant characterization in respect to total porosity, pore size and interconnectivity, histograms and new bone formation quantification. The distribution of *de novo* bone formed in the explants can be assessed and 3D visualized using image processing software (e.g. CT Analyser and ANT 3D creator).

Histological analysis

After μ-CT analysis, the explants are further processed as follows:

- Harvest implants after each implantation time.
- Remove tissues around the implants with sterile plastic tweezers.
- Immerse the implants in a PBS solution.

- Explants are decalcified in K-CX solution.
- Fix the implants with 10% formalin neutral buffered saline solution for about 90 min.
- Dehydration of the explants in an ascending series grade ethanol/water solution (from 90–100%) for 19 hr, followed by washing three times with xylene.
- Soak the explants in paraffin at 62°C and allow to solidify at −5°C.
- Prepare sections with a thickness of 5 μm using a microtome.
- Mount the slices in a micro-slide glass.
- Paraffin should be removed by placing the slides in the oven at 71°C for 20 min and allowed to let cool down at RT.
- Remove the remnant paraffin from slides by immersion in hexane for 5 min and subsequently in an ethylene/propylene mixture for 3 min.
- Soak the slides three times in 100% ethanol for 2 min each time of immersion.
- Transfer the slides to 90% ethanol and then to 70% and wash with tap water.
- Stain with H&E staining.

Quantification of calcium (extraction of calcium from explants)

- Explants are washed with Ca and Mg-free PBS solution.
- Transfer to a 2 mL Eppendorf.
- Add 0.2 mL of 1 N HCl solution per explant.
- Agitate in an orbital shaker to extract calcium for the period of 12 hr.
- Centrifuge at 15 000 rpm for 10 min.
- Supernatants are assayed (o-cresolphthalein complexation color development method) using a commercial calcium assay kit (Calcium C-test™).

   Note: Calcium content is determined by measuring the absorbance at 570 nm. Experiments are carried out in triplicate using 3 replicates per experimental condition (n = 9).

Characterization

In vivo studies

- Micro-CT analysis revealed that SPCL scaffolds seeded with rBMSCs cultured with Dex-loaded CMCht/PAMAM nanoparticles induced the formation of new bone (white areas) after 4 weeks of subcutaneous implantation in the back of F344/N rats (Fig. 2).
- From histological studies (Fig. 3), we observed no signs of infection or acute inflammatory reaction at the implantation sites for all implants after 4 weeks of implantation.
- No bone formation in the explants of SPCL alone (control) and SPCL scaffolds seeded with RBMSCs cultured in both MEM and Dex was observed (Figs. 3A–3C).
- From histological analysis, it is evident that the massive area of high attenuation (white area) observed by micro-CT corresponds to new bone formed (back arrow, Fig. 3D).

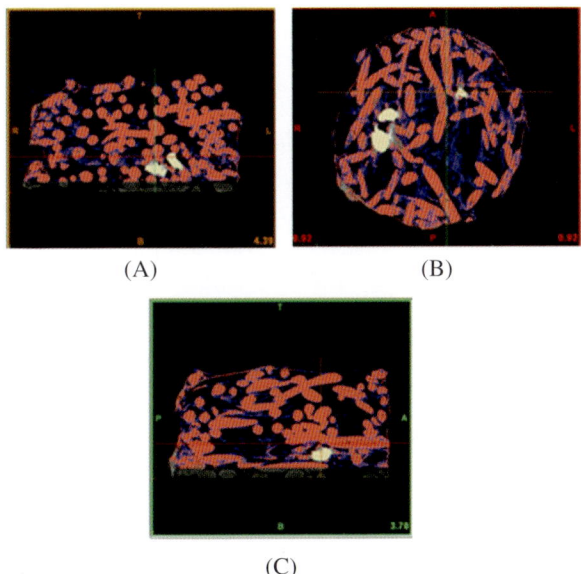

(A)   (B)

(C)

Fig. 2 2D micro-CT images of the rBMSCs/SPCL explants (4 weeks of implantation) in which cells were pre-cultured with Dex-loaded CMCht/PAMAM dendrimer nanoparticles prior to implantation. White regions correspond to *de novo* bone formation.

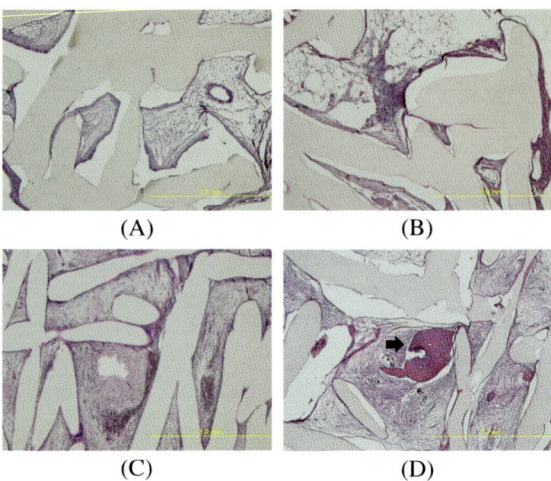

Fig. 3 Photomicrographs from H&E histological sections of explants (4 weeks of implantation): SPCL explants (A), RBMSCs/SPCL explants (B), RBMSCs/SPCL explants with cells treated with Dex from culture medium prior implantation (C), and RBMSCs/SPCL explants with cells pre-cultured with Dex-loaded CMCht/PAMAM dendrimer nanoparticles prior implantation (D). Black arrow indicates new bone formed.

- The superior osteogenesis (*de novo* bone formation) in the explants whose RBMSCs were supplemented with Dex-loaded CMCht/PAMAM dendrimer nanoparticles as compared to those whose RBMSCs were supplemented with Dex from culture media is the most important achievement in this study.

References

1. JM Oliveira, RA Sousa, N Kotobuki, *et al.* (2009) The osteogenic differentiation of rat bone marrow stromal cells cultured with dexamethasone-loaded carboxymethylchitosan/poly(amidoamine) dendrimer nanoparticles. *Biomaterials* **30**(5): 804–813.
2. JM Oliveira, RA Sousa, PB Malafaya, *et al.* (2011) *In vivo* study of dendron-like nanoparticles for stem cells tune-up: From nano to tissues. *Nanomedicine: Nanotechnology, Biology, and Medicine* **7**: 914–924.

1

Protocol for Osteogenesis of BMSC in Calcium Phosphate Ceramics

Eui Kyun Park,[*,‡]*
Hong-In Shin,[*]*
Shin-Yoon Kim[†]*,*
and Jiwon Lim[*]*

[*]Department of Pathology and Regenerative Medicine, School of Dentistry, Kyungpook National University, Daegu 700-412 Korea.
[†]Department of Orthopaedic Surgery, School of Medicine, Kyungpook National University, Daegu 700-412 Korea.

Background

- Bone tissue provides mechanical support to the body and a stem cell reservoir for blood cells. Defects in bone tissue can be resulted by variety of causes such as trauma, cancer and necrosis, and may lead to life-threatening consequences. Effective treatment of large bone lesion requires biocompatible materials for mechanical support and enhanced regeneration by host bone.

- Tissue engineering technology using three-dimensional scaffold and autologous or allogeneic stem cells is a promising treatment method for a large bone lesion.

- Among currently available scaffolds, calcium phosphate ceramics have been widely used for bone defects because they provide mechanical support as well as growth of neighboring host bone into the defected area. They also have excellent biocompatibility and biodegradability.[1]

- Among commonly used stem cells, BMSCs have attracted great interest for bone regeneration because these cells are capable of differentiating into various types of cells, including osteoblasts.

- In addition, hBMSCs can be easily expanded over several subcultures maintaining their stem cell potentials, and differentiated into osteoblasts in response to osteogenic cocktail (50 µg/mL α-ascorbic acid, 10 mM β-glycerophosphate and 100 nM dexamethasone).

- Osteoblast differentiation of human BMSCs can be assessed by cytological stainings such as Alizarin Red S and von Kossa, and molecular evaluation of osteoblast marker genes including collagen, type I, osteocalcin and bone sialoprotein by reverse transcriptase polymerase chain reaction.

Culturing Methods for Human BMSCs

- Collect bone marrow aspirate (8–10 mL) in a heparin tube (The heparinized bone marrow aspirate can be kept for several hours at 4°C).

- To isolate BMSCs, bone marrow aspirate should be carefully laid over histopaque 1077 solution, and spun 400×g for 30 min.

- Collect mononuclear cell layer and then wash cells twice with PBS, pH 7.4.
- Re-suspend the bone marrow mononuclear cells in α-MEM containing 10% FBS and incubate at 37°C in a humidified atmosphere of 5% CO_2 for 24–48 hr.
- Remove the non-adherent cells and expand the adherent cells for further experiments. The isolated human BMSCs show fibroblast-like and spindle-shaped morphological features (Fig. 1).

Characterization of BMSCs

- Using flow cytometry, cell surface cluster of differentiation (CD) can be analyzed. BMSCs are positive for cell surface markers such as CD29, CD44, CD49a, CD71, CD73, CD90, CD105, CD146, CD166, CD271, and STRO-1, but negative for CD14 or CD34 (Fig. 2 and Table 1).

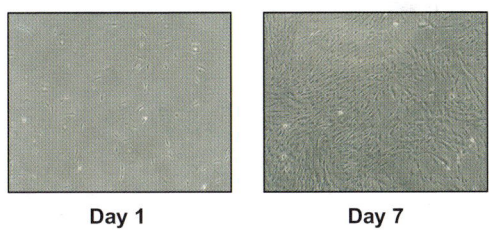

Day 1   **Day 7**

Fig. 1 Morphological features of primary hBMSCs. (Original magnification × 40.)

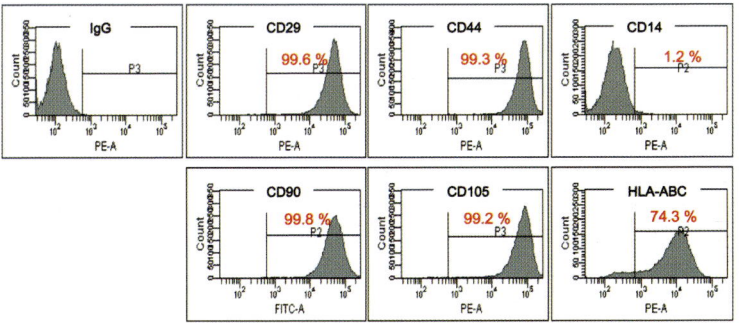

Fig. 2 Cell surface typing of hBMSCs with some mesenchymal stem cell markers.

Table 1 Cell surface typing of hBMSCs isolated by several donors.

MSC markers	Donors					
	1	2	3	4	5	6
CD29	96.8	99.9	98.9	96.6	99.7	99.2
CD44	96.9	99.4	99.7	96.3	99.6	99.3
CD90	96.9	99.9	99.7	96.4	99.8	98
CD105	97.4	99.9	99.5	97.0	99.5	99.4
CD146	37.8	90.1	76.1	81.1	42.8	49.6
HLA-ABC	97.2	98.9	98.6	97.0	99.7	87.3
CD14	1.5	2.4	0.8	2.0	2.6	2
CD34	0.6	0.5	0.2	1.2	0.3	0.5

Preparation of Calcium Phosphate Scaffold

- To obtain calcium metaphosphate (CMP) and hydroxyapatite (HAp) powders, heat calcium phosphate monohydrate [$Ca(H_2PO_4)_2 \cdot H_2O$] and tribasic calcium phosphate [$Ca_3(PO_4)_2$] at 670°C for 578 hr.
- To obtain fine ground slurry, CMP and HA powders can beZrO_2 ball-milled and the slurry needs to be dried in a rotary vacuum evaporator and ground again with an agate mortar.
- Press-form CMP and HA disks with a 15 mm diameter and a 1.5 mm thickness.
- Sinter all specimens at 890°C for 3 hr (Fig. 3).
- Porous CMP scaffold can be fabricated via a polymeric sponge method. The paste for coating is prepared by mixing the powders with distilled water at a 25:75 ratio in vol% with 5 wt% PVA (polyvinylalcohol), polycarbonic ammonium, and a drying control chemical additive. Polyurethane sponges are immersed in the prepared pastes, and the

coated specimens can be dried at room temperature for 6 hr and then sintered at a multi-step heating schedule; 600°C at 2°C/min to burn out the organic components and then sintered at 890°C at 5°C/min for 3 hr. The porous CMP samples are machined into the desired dimensions (Fig. 3).

Analysis for Osteogenesis *In Vitro* and *In Vivo*

- Alkaline phosphatase activity or staining.
- Alizarin Red S and von Kossa staining for mineralization (calcium precipitation).
- H&E staining for bone formation and maturation (mature bone has lacunae and osteocyte resides in the lacunae).
- Expression of osteogenesis marker genes such as collagen type I, bone sialoprotein, alkaline phosphatase and osteocalcin using real time or conventional RT-PCR.
- *In vivo* bone formation analysis. In order to analyze *in vivo* effect of scaffold seeded with human BMSCs on bone regeneration, calvarial defect model of BALB/c-nu nude mouse can be used. CMP porous disk (5 mm diameter and 0.5 mm thickness) needs to be seeded with human BMSCs (1.2×10^6 cells/scaffold) and cultured in α-MEM containing 10% FBS and antibiotics. Next day, using dental trephine, a hole in calvariun with diameter of 5 mm can be made and porous

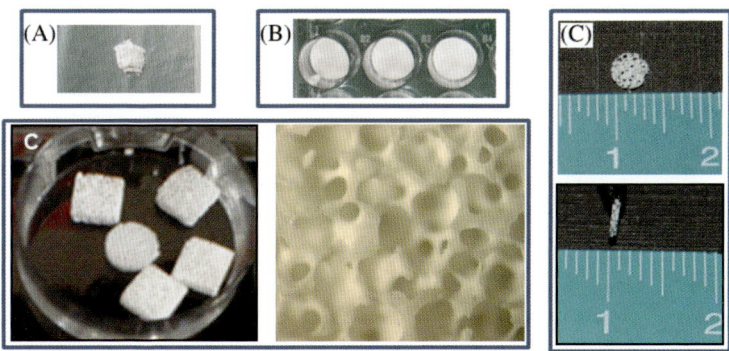

Fig. 3 Stereoscopic view of (A) powder, (B) compress-formed disks in a 24-well culture plate, (C) porous 3D disk and (D) blocks and porous disk of CMP.

CMP disk combined with human BMSCs are implanted in the calvarial defect (Fig. 4). After 4–10 weeks of implantation, bone regeneration in the calvaria can be assessed by H&E and trichrome stainings and by measuring the bone marker gene expression.

Requirements

Minimum Essential Medium (α-MEM), antibiotics (100 unit/mL penicillin and 100 µg/mL streptomycin), PBS, Trypsin-EDTA, FBS, CMP and HA scaffolds. HA and CMP disks, porous CMP scaffolds.

Characterization

- Stimulation of osteoblast differentiation of hBMSCs cultured on HAp and CMP disk stained with ALP showed ALP-positive cells on the CMP disk were increased compared with culture plate and HAp disk, suggesting that CMP stimulates osteoblast differentiation of human BMSCs.
- Consistent with ALP staining, expression of osteoblast differentiation markers were also increased in BMSCs cultured on CMP disk compared to those on HAp disk or culture plate.
- Porous CMP could support osteoblast differentiation *in vitro* as assessed by ALP staining and marker expression (Fig. 5).
- Implantation of porous CMP disk seeded with hBMSCs into calvarial defect in nude mice showed enhanced bone regeneration as shown by H&E staining (Fig. 6).
- These results demonstrate that CMP scaffold combined with hBMSCs enhances osteoblast differentiation *in vitro* and thus bone regeneration *in vivo*.

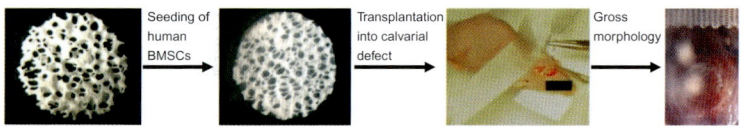

Fig. 4 Procedure of calvarial implantation of CMP disk seeded with human BMSCs.

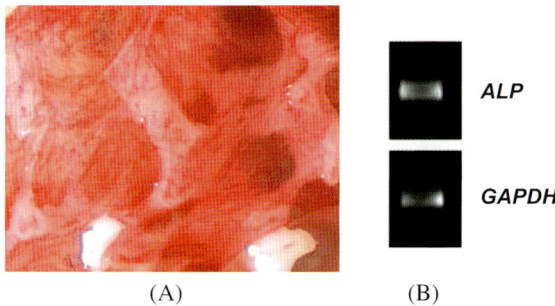

(A)   (B)

Fig. 5   ALP staining (A) and expression of osteoblast marker genes (B) in human BMSCs cultured on porous CMP scaffold.

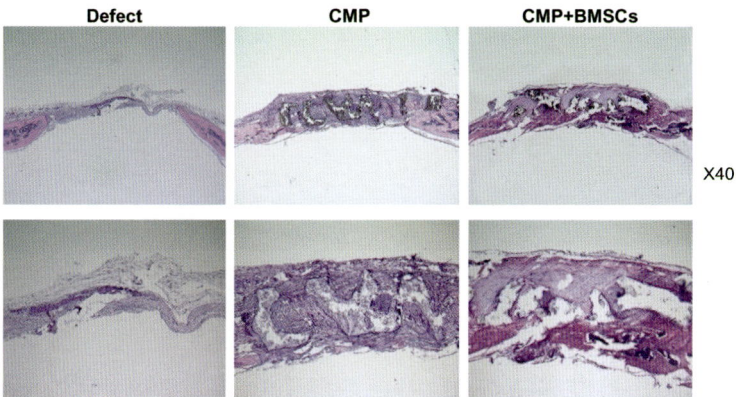

Fig. 6   H&E staining of calvarial bone after 8 weeks of implantation of CMP-hBMSCs (magnification of ×40 and ×100 was shown).

Reference

1.   EK Park, YE Lee, JY Choi, *et al.* (2004) Cellular biocompatibility and stimulatory effects of calcium metaphosphate on osteoblastic differentiation of human bone marrow-derived stromal cells. *Biomaterials* **25**(17): 3403–3411.

J

Protocol of Osteoblastic Differentiation of BMSC in Biodegradable Scaffolds Composed of Gelatin and β-Tricalcium Phosphate

Masaya Yamamoto and Yasuhiko Tabata

Department of Biomaterials, Institute for Frontier Medical Sciences, Kyoto University, 53 Kawara-cho Shogoin, Sakyo-ku, Kyoto 606-8507, Japan.

Background

- Bone tissue engineering has attracted much attention as an alternative method to restore bone defects. Indeed, it is possible to obtain osteoblasts from the periosteum and/or bone explants. However, it is difficult to isolate osteoblasts from patients due to the shortage of donor sites. Therefore, MSCs have been extensively investigated as a potential cell source for bone tissue engineering, because MSCs can be easily harvested from bone marrow or adipose tissue of patients, proliferate well in culture, and differentiate into osteoblasts under the appropriate culture condition.

- Osteogenic growth factors or some glucocorticoids have been shown to induce the osteoblast differentiation of MSCs *in vitro*. Upon culturing on a tissue culture dish in the presence of dexamethasone, MSCs form the bone nodule of 3-dimension containing bone-like mineralized ECM in concert with osteoblast differentiation. Therefore, the bone-like 3-D milieu plays an important role in the osteoblast differentiation of MSCs.

- It has been demonstrated that scaffolds function as an artificial 3-D milieu of bone cells in bone tissue engineering. In this chapter, biodegradable scaffolds composed of gelatin and β-tricalcium phosphate (β-TCP) are investigated as an artificial 3-dimensional milieu to induce osteoblast differentiation of MSCs.[1]

Fabrication of Biodegradable Scaffolds Composed of Gelatin and β-TCP

- Mix 3 wt% aqueous solution of gelatin containing 3 wt% β-TCP at 5000 rpm at 37°C for 3 min by using a homogenizer (ED-12, Nihonseiki Co., Tokyo, Japan).

- Add 0.16 wt% of an aqueous solution of glutaraldehyde to the foamy solution and further mix for 15 sec with the homogenizer.

- Cast the resulting foamy solution into a polypropylene dish of 138 × 138 cm^2 and 5 mm depth, followed by leaving at 4°C for 12 hr for gelatin cross-linking.

- Place the freeze-dried scaffold in 100 mM aqueous glycine solution at 37°C for 1 hr to block the residual aldehyde groups of glutaraldehyde.
- Wash the scaffold with double distilled water and freeze-dry, followed by cutting into cubes of $5 \times 5 \times 5$ mm^3.

Isolation of BMSC

- Harvest femurs and tibias from legs of Fischer rat (female, 3 weeks old).
- Flush the marrow cavity with 1 mL of PBS using 22 gauge syringes into a tube with PBS.
- Plate bone marrow suspension onto a tissue culture dish, followed by maintaining in DMEM supplemented with 15 vol% FCS and 1% antibiotics under a humidified atmosphere of 5% CO_2 at 37°C.
- Remove the non-adherent hematopoietic cells 3 days later by washing with the culture media and culture the adherent spindle-shaped MSC for 7 days. Change the medium every 2–3 days.
- Subculture at 80–90% of confluence to expand MSC for cell seeding.

Cell Culture of Cell-Seeded Gelatin Scaffolds Incorporating β-TCP

- Place 500 μl of cell suspension (2×10^6 cells/mL) and the scaffold in 5 mL tubes with 12 mm of inner diameter (2236-012, I waki Glass Co. Ltd., Chiba, Japan) and agitate the tube on an orbital shaker at 300 rpm for 6 hr to facilitate cell seeding (Fig. 1).

Table 1 Characterization of gelatin scaffolds incorporating β-TCP.

β-TCP content (wt%)	Pore size (μm)	Porosity (%)	Compression modulus (MPa)
0	184.9 ± 58.2	96.6	0.27 ± 0.01
50	179.1 ± 27.8	95.9	1.13 ± 0.13

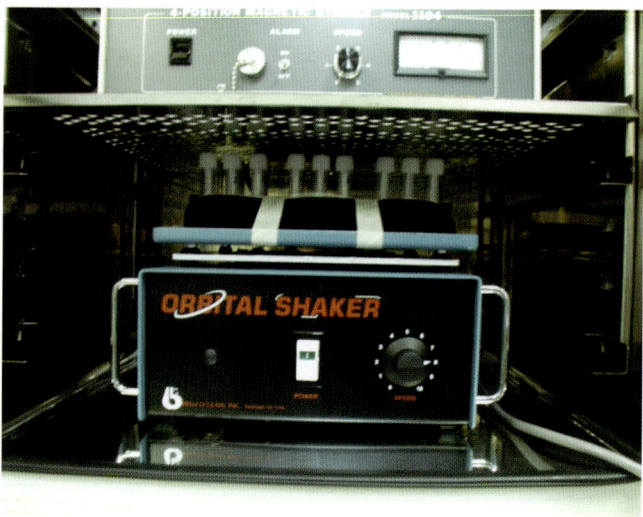

Fig. 1   Agitated cell seeding into scaffolds using an orbital shaker.

- Wash the MSC-seeded scaffold with PBS to exclude non-adherent cells.
- Maintaining the cell-seeded scaffold in DMEM supplemented with 15 vol% FCS, 10 nM dexamethasone, 50 µg/mL ascorbic acid, and 10 mM β-glycerophosphate (osteoblast differentiation medium) at 37°C in a 5% CO_2–95% air atmosphere.
- Spire six of the cell-seeded scaffold by one needle and maintain them in the spinner flasks (1965-00100, Bellco Glass, Inc.) at the stirring rate of 50 rpm with 150 mL of osteoblast differentiation medium (Fig. 2).
- Refresh the medium every 3 days.

Analysis for Osteoblast Differentiation *In Vitro*

- SEM observation for osteoblast adhesion on the pore surface of scaffolds (Fig. 3).
- DNA assay for cell growth (Fig. 4).
- Alkaline phosphatase (ALP) activity assay for osteoblast differentiation (Fig. 5A).
- ELISA for osteocalcin contents (Fig. 5B).
- H&E staining for bone-like tissue formation in scaffolds (Fig. 6).

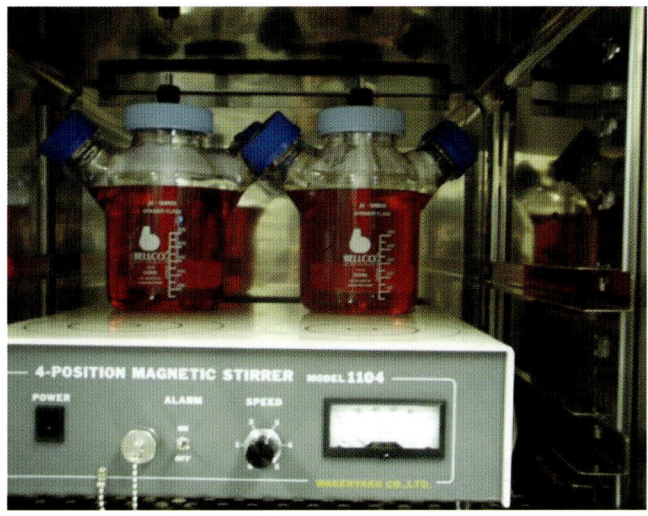

Fig. 2   Stirring cell culture using spinner flasks.

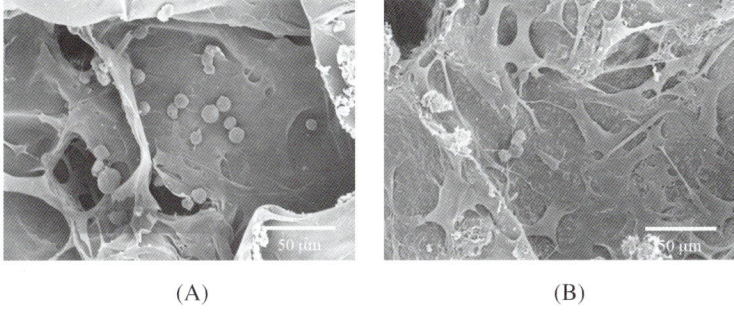

(A)   (B)

Fig. 3   SEM of MSC attached to gelatin scaffolds incorporating (A) 0 and (B) 50 wt% of β-TCP 6 hr after cell seeding. The number of cells applied is 5×10^6 cells/sponge.

Requirements

DMEM (low glucose), β-glycerophosphate, ascorbic acid, dexamethasone, antibiotics (100 unit/mL penicillin and 100 μg/mL streptomycin), PBS, trypsin-EDTA, FCS, syringes (22 gauge), orbital shaker, spinner flasks, cell culture wares, and spectrophotometer (UV/VIS microplate reader).

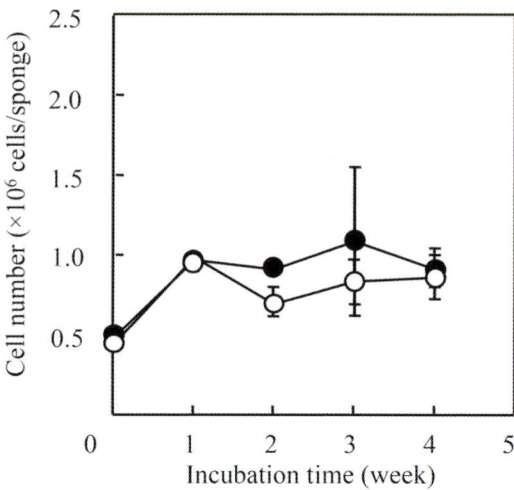

Fig. 4 Time course of MSC proliferation in the gelatin sponges incorporating 0 (○) and 50 (●) of β-TCP by the stirring culture method.

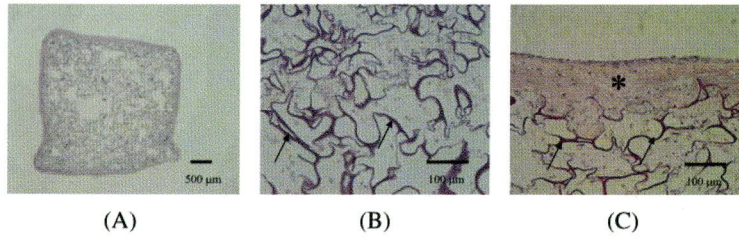

(A)   (B)   (C)

Fig. 5 Histological cross-sections of MSCs attached to gelatin scaffolds incorporating 50 wt% of β-TCP after 4 weeks of culture in the osteoblast medium. The scale bar measures 500 μm in (A) full cross-section and 100 μm (B, C) in higher magnification views of (B) center and (C) periphery in the scaffold. Arrows indicate the residual gelatin scaffold incorporating β-TCP. Asterisks indicate the bone newly formed.

Characterization

- When seeded into the scaffold by an agitated method, MSCs were homogeneously distributed throughout the scaffold. The morphology of cells attached on the scaffold with β-TCP got more spindle than those without β-TCP (Figs. 3 and 5).

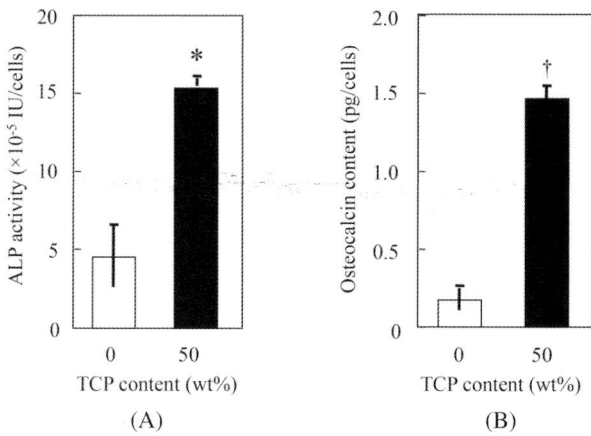

Fig. 6 (A) ALP activity and (B) osteocalcin content of MSCs in scaffolds incorporating 0 (white) and 50 (black) of β-TCP 2 and 4 weeks after culture in the osteoblast differentiation medium, respectively. *p < 0.05; significant against the ALP activity of MSCs cultured in the scaffold without β-TCP. †p < 0.05; significant against the osteocalcin content of MSCs in the scaffold without β-TCP.

- The *in vitro* proliferation and differentiation of MSCs was influenced by the incorporation ratio of β-TCP in the scaffold (Figs. 4 and 6).
- MSCs were homogeneously distributed and proliferated in the inner portion of the scaffold, although new bone was not formed. Significant bone formation was observed at the peripheral portion of gelatin scaffold (Fig. 5).
- We concluded that the attachment, proliferation, and osteoblast differentiation of MSCs were influenced by scaffold composition of gelatin and β-TCP.

Notes

- Gelatin scaffolds prepared have an interconnected pore structure with an average pore size of 180 μm, irrespective of the β-TCP content. The stiffness of the scaffold became higher with an increase in the content of β-TCP.
- The gelatin-β-TCP scaffold can be readily cut by a scalpel to formulate in different shapes.

- The amount of β-TCP incorporated can be controlled by changing the weight ratio of gelatin and β-TCP in the scaffold.

- Simple foaming of gelatin solution permitted to prepare the gelatin scaffold of sponge structure not only to facilitate *in vitro* cell seeding but also to function as the release carrier for growth factor. The release profile of growth factors could be readily changed by altering the cross-linking extent of gelatin in scaffold preparation, while the growth factor release contributes to the enhancement of growth factor activity *in vivo*.[2]

References

1. Y Takahashi, M Yamamoto, Y Tabata. (2005) Osteogenic differentiation of mesenchymal stem cells in biodegradable sponges composed of gelatin and β-tricalcium phosphate. *Biomaterials* **26**(17): 3587–3596.

2. Y Takahashi, M Yamamoto, Y Tabata. (2005) Enhanced osteoinduction by controlled release of bone morphogenetic protein-2 from biodegradable sponge composed of gelatin and β-tricalcium phosphate. *Biomaterials* **26**(23): 4856–4865.

K

Protocol of Cardiomyogenic Induction of hMSCs on Dendrimer-Immobilized Surfaces Displaying with D-Glucose

*Mee-Hae Kim and Masahiro Kino-oka**

---

*Department of Biotechnology, Graduate School of Engineering, Osaka University, 2-1 Yamadaoka, Suita, Osaka 565-0871, Japan.

Background

- BMSCs are a population of self-renewing, multipotent cells which have significant clinical potential for cellular therapies and tissue engineering. These cells are able to differentiate into several committed phenotypes including osteogenic, chondrogenic, adipogenic, cardiomyogenic, and neurogenic lineages when appropriately stimulated. However, one of the limitations of using MSCs for clinical applications is their low differentiation efficiency. The differentiation pathways of MSCs are highly regulated by intrinsic and extrinsic signals in their niches.

- Cell morphology regulates the switch in lineage commitment of BMSCs by modulating endogenous Rho family GTPase activities. BMSCs that adhere, flatten and spread undergo osteogenesis, while those that do not spread and are round become adipocytes. Changes in cell morphology activate signal transduction pathways that involve the main elements of Rho family GTPases and downstream signaling molecules. This finding suggests that extracellular signals can be locally integrated by the endogenous Rho family GTPases to coordinate dynamic cytoskeletal rearrangements that are necessary for directing the fates of stem cells.

- Dendrimer-immobilized surfaces displaying D-glucose have been shown to play an important role with respect to the function and morphological changes of stem cells. If BMSCs are cultured on a dendrimer-immobilized surface, they start to differentiate down a cardiomyogenic pathway.

- We differentiated BMSCs into cardiomyocyte-like cells on dendrimer-immobilized surfaces displaying D-glucose.

BMSC Culture

- MSCs were expanded for an appropriate time in DMEM supplemented with 10% FBS and antibiotics.
- The seeding density was 5.0×10^3 viable cells/cm^2.
- On day 3 of culture, the spent medium was replaced with fresh medium.

- The number of viable cells was estimated using trypan blue exclusion and a hemacytometer.
- At 70% confluence, cells were detached using 0.1% trypsin/0.02% EDTA solution. Cells cultured for less than 5 passages were used in subsequent experiments.

Preparation of Dendrimer-Immobilized Surfaces Displaying D-Glucose

- The dendrimer surface was prepared using conventional 8-well tissue culture-grade PS plates. A fifth-generation (G5) surface was created by changing the generation number of synthesized dendrimers over four reactions. This was conducted under sterile conditions as outlined in Fig. 1.
- Step 1: To display a hydroxyl group on the starter surface, an aqueous solution of 50 μmol/mL potassium *tert*-butoxide (*tert*-BuOK) was poured into each well, followed by 1 hr

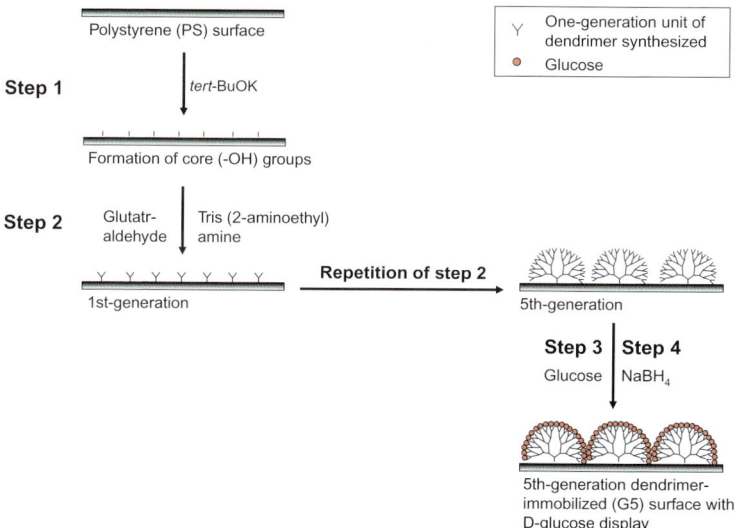

Fig. 1 A schematic illustrating the procedure we used to prepare a G5 dendrimer-immobilized surface displaying D-glucose.

incubation at ambient temperature. The well was then washed 3 times with sterilized water.

- Step 2: An aqueous solution of 360 µmol/mL glutaraldehyde was introduced into the well and allowed to stand for 1 hr, followed by washing with a large amount of water. The well was treated with 360 µmol/mL tris(2-aminoethyl) amine solution (pH 9.0) for 1 hr to produce a dendron structure and then rinsed with water. Step 2 was repeated until the fifth-generation surface was synthesized.
- Step 3: To display D-glucose as a terminal ligand, 0.5 µmol/mL D-glucose solution was added to the well and allowed to stand for 2 hr.
- Step 4: A 0.5 µmol/mL sodium borohydride solution was poured into the well and left to stand for 24 hr. The well was washed with water, yielding a G5 dendrimer surface displaying D-glucose.

Characterization of BMSCs

- To confirm phenotypes and differentiation capacities of hMSCs cultured on the dendrimer surfaces for 7 days, immunostaining for an undifferentiated MSC surface marker and several mesenchymal lineage-specific markers were conducted.
- Cells were fixed with 4% paraformaldehyde, and permeabilized with 0.25% Triton X-100 in PBS for 4 min.
- Non-specific proteins were masked by incubating in Block Ace for 15 min at ambient temperature.
- Cells were then incubated with a primary antibody at 4°C overnight.
- We used mouse primary antibodies against CD105 (endoglin), desmin, fast skeletal myosin heavy chain (fast skeletal MHC), α-smooth muscle actin (α-SMA) or cardiac troponin T (cTnT).
- Cells were washed with Tris-buffered saline (TBS), and then incubated with Alexa Fluor 488-conjugated anti-rabbit or anti-mouse immunoglobulin G (IgG) for 1 hr.
- TOPRO-3 was used to stain for F-actin and nuclei. Digital images were obtained using a confocal laser-scanning microscope through ×60 and ×100 objective lenses.

Morphological change in BMSCs Cultured on a G5 Surface

- Observation of cells on day 3 of culture revealed that most of those cells on the G5 surface were round. Those on the PS surface showed stretched morphologies. On day 7, cells on the G5 surface formed loosely attached aggregates, while those on the PS surface formed flatter and confluent monolayers that were firmly attached to the surface. (Fig. 2)

Phenotypes and Differentiation Capacities of BMSCs

- Immunostaining for the MSC surface marker CD105 (endoglin) revealed that nearly all of the cells cultured on PS surface were CD105-positive. Cells cultured on G5 surface were completely negative for this marker (Fig. 3b1).

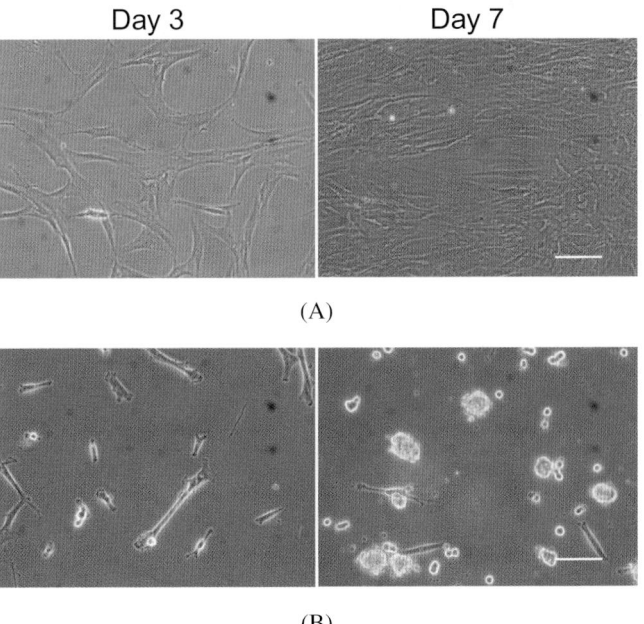

Fig. 2   Phase contrast images of hMSCs cultured on PS (A) and G5 (B) surfaces. The scale bars indicate 100 μm.

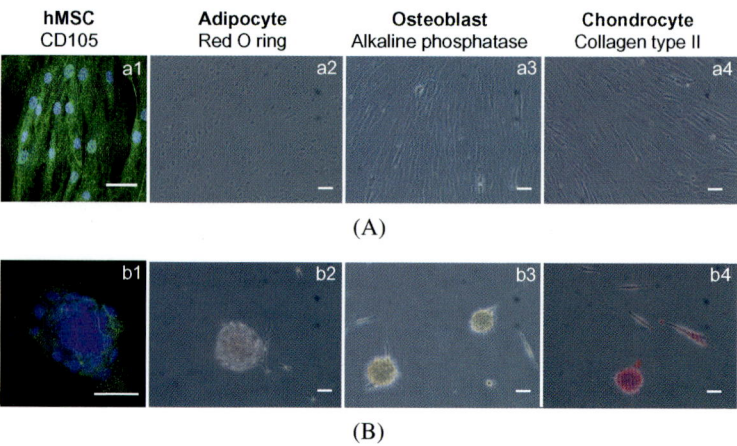

(A)

(B)

Fig. 3 Immunocytochemical detection of MSC surface marker and mesenchymal lineage-specific markers in hMSCs cultured on (A) PS and (B) G5 surface. Images were obtained on day 7, and scale bars indicate 100 μm.

- With respect to lineage-specific differentiation markers, cells cultured on all surfaces were negative for osteoblast (Figs. 3a2 and 3b2) and adipocyte markers (Figs. 3a3 and 3b3). The chondrocyte marker collagen type II was observed around aggregated cells on the G5 surface (Fig. 3b4).

Characterization of Cardiomyogenic Differentiation

- To identify induction of different myogenic lineages (cardiac, skeletal and smooth muscle cells), we assessed protein expression of markers for these specific lineages (Fig. 4).
- Expression of fast skeletal MHC and cTnT, markers of skeletal muscle cells and cardiomyocytes, respectively, were not detected in cells cultured on the PS surface (Figs. 4a1 and 4a2). These markers were obvious in cells grown and differentiated on the G5 surface (Figs. 4b1 and 4b2). Fast skeletal MHC expression was restricted to the peripheral regions of aggregated cells on the G5 surface. Expression of cTnT was abundant in cells grown on the G5 surface (Fig. 4b2).

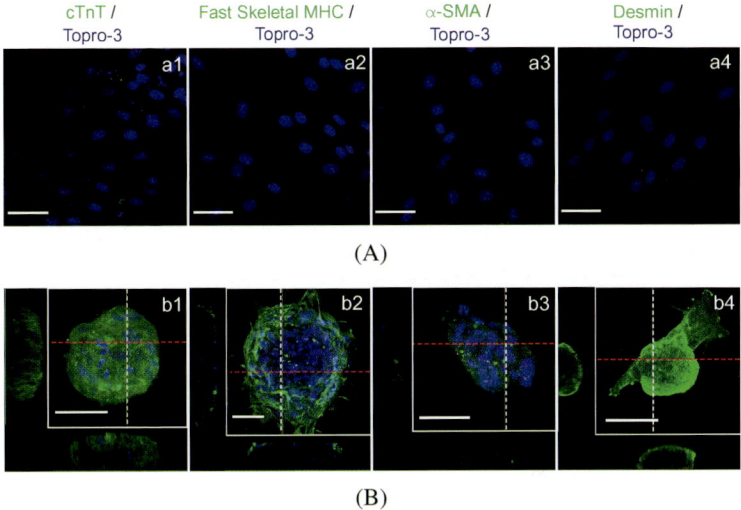

Fig. 4 Immunostaining results showing nuclei (blue) and desmin (green), α-SMA (green), fast skeletal MHC (green) or cTnT (green) in hMSCs cultured on (A) PS and (B) G5 surfaces. The images at the bottom and on the right for b1, b2, b3 and b4 show images sectioned along the x-z (dotted white lines) and y-z (dotted red lines) planes. Images were acquired on day 7. The scale bars show 50 μm.

- α-SMA, a specific marker of smooth muscle cells, was expressed at lower intensity in cells cultured on both the PS and G5 surfaces (Figs. 4a3 and 4a4).
- These results demonstrate that hMSCs cultured on the G5 surface aggregate to a greater extent, while at the same time inducing the cardiomyogenic phenotype as shown by the abundant expression of cTnT.

Notes

- It is possible to induce BMSCs to follow a cardiomyogenic fate in the absence of additional differentiation factors.
- The prepared dendrimer surfaces were stored at 4°C under sterile conditions until use for no more than 2 weeks before they were used.

References

1. M-H Kim, M Kino-oka, M Nao, *et al.* (2010) Cardiomyogenic induction of human mesenchymal stem cells by altered Rho family GTPase expression on dendrimer-immobilized surface with D-glucose display. *Biomaterials* **33**: 7666–7677.
2. M-H Kim, M Kino-oka, M Taya. (2010) Designing culture surfaces based on cell anchoring mechanisms to regulate cell morphologies and functions. *Biotechnology Advance* **28**: 7–16.

L

Protocol of Cardiomyocyte Differentiation of BMSC by Small Molecules

Ki-Chul Hwang, Woochul Chang, and Byeong-Wook Song

Cardiovascular Research Institute, Yonsei University College of Medicine, 250 Seongsanno, Seodaemun-gu, Seoul, 120-752, Korea.

Background

- Because the intrinsic repair mechanism of the heart is insufficient, which results in a considerable loss of cardiomyocytes, regenerated cardiomyocytes could be a useful tool for transplantation to ischemic heart.

- MSCs have become one of the most potentiated cell sources for repairing infarcted myocardium because MSCs are multipotent cells capable of differentiating into cardiac myocytes, endothelial cells, and vascular smooth muscle cells both *in vivo* and *in vitro* under the appropriate culture conditions.

- Stem cell fate is determined by intrinsic regulators and/or the extracellular environment. Stem cell differentiation is generally controlled by growing the cells in a specific extracellular environment with growth factors as well as genetic manipulations. However, most of these conditions are either incompletely defined or non-specific in regulating the desired cellular process.

- Protein kinases, the members of a large family of proteins involved in modulating many known signaling pathways, are likely to play important roles in regulating stem cell differentiation programs because important bio-processes such as cell fate are likely to be determined by an elaborate orchestration of multiple signaling pathways. In addition, cell permeable small molecules to modulate activation of protein kinase have several merits, including the ability for temporal, tunable and modular control of specific protein function.

- Since cardiomyogenic differentiation of MSCs is likely to be controlled by a complicated orchestration of many signaling pathways, signal modulators such as protein kinases are likely to play important role in balancing multiple signals involved in differentiation. Recent study demonstrated that protein kinase C (PKC) regulated the cardiac differentiation of stem cells.

- Therefore, research efforts focused on the search for a chemical reagent and mechanism that regulates systematic differentiation of MSCs. We introduced the cardiomyogenic differentiation of MSCs using PKC activator affected PKC signaling pathway.

Isolation and Culture of MSCs

- Isolate from the femoral and tibia bones of 4-weeks-old male Sprague-Dawley rats.
- Flush the bone marrow with 10 mL of DMEM-low glucose, supplemented with 10% FBS and 1% antibiotic-penicillin and streptomycin.
- Recover mononuclear cells from the interface after centrifugation in Percoll and wash to 10% DMEM twice.
- Re-suspend the collected cell in 10% FBS-DMEM and plate in flasks at 10^6 cells per 100 cm^2.
- Maintain cells at 37°C in a humidified atmosphere containing 5% CO_2.
- Discard the non-adherent hematopoietic cells after 48–72 hours, add fresh complete medium, and replace every 3 or 4 days for approximately 10 days.
- Subculture when these primary MSCs reached 80–90% of confluence and use the MSCs passage 2 or 3 times.

MSCs Characterization

- Characterize properties of MSC by immunocytochemistry or FACS using positive or negative marker of MSCs.
- MSCs lacked CD14 and CD34 as negative isotype control whereas they were positively stained CD71, CD90, CD105, CD106 and intracellular adhesion molecule (ICAM)-1 through immunocytochemistry or FACS (Fig. 1).

Analysis for Cardiomyogenic Differentiation *In Vitro*

- Morphological analysis compared with neonatal rat ventricular cardiomyocytes.
- Immunocytochemistry for morphological change comparison.
- Sandwich ELISA for cardiac-specific characteristics of differentiated cardiomyogenic cells.

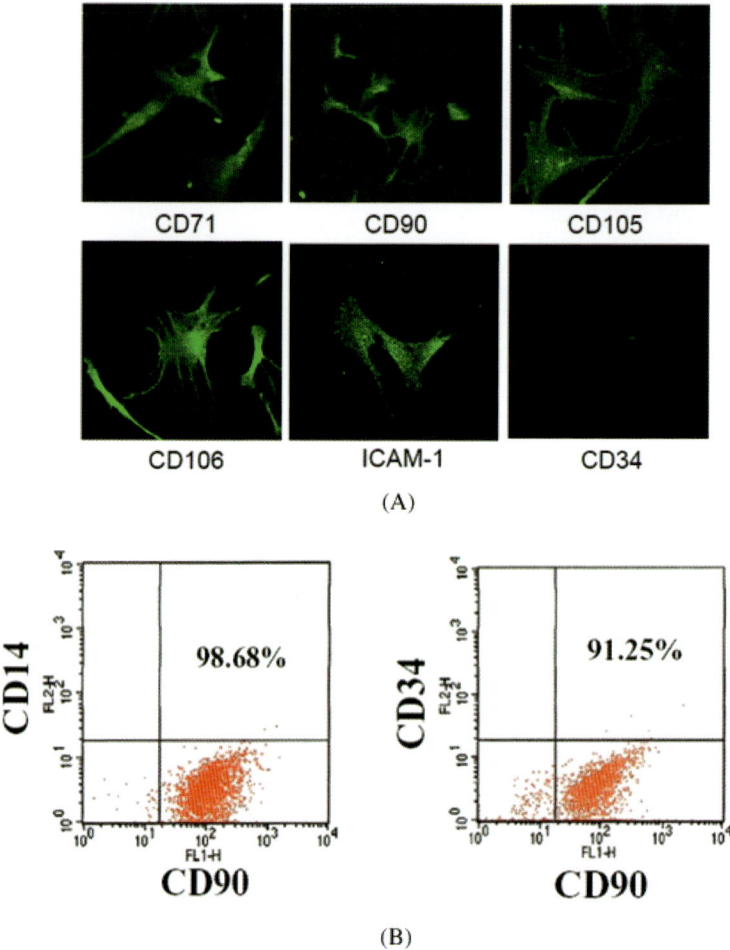

Fig. 1 Characterization of MSCs. (A) Immunocytochemistry; (B) FACS Calibur system (magnification ×400)

- RT-PCR for expression level of alpha-, beta-adrenergic receptor and muscarinic receptor and calcium handling-related protein.
- Immunoblot analysis for hypertrophic response in cardiomyogenic cells.

Requirements

Sprague-Dawley rats (8 weeks), DMEM (low glucose), antibiotics (100 unit/mL penicillin and 100 µg/mL streptomycin), PBS, trypsin-EDTA, FBS, PKC activator, antibody (cardiac specific marker: cardiac troponin T, myosin light chain, myosin heavy chain, NK2 transcription factor-related, locus 5, Myocyte-specific enhancer factor 2) and NE (norepinephrine).

Characterization

• Cardiomyogenic differentiation was modulated by PKC family (Fig. 2).
• After 9 days of culture with PKC activator, MSCs had a myocyte-like morphology (Fig. 3).
• In sandwich ELISA, the expression of cardiac specific marker was highly regulated about 9 days (Fig. 4).

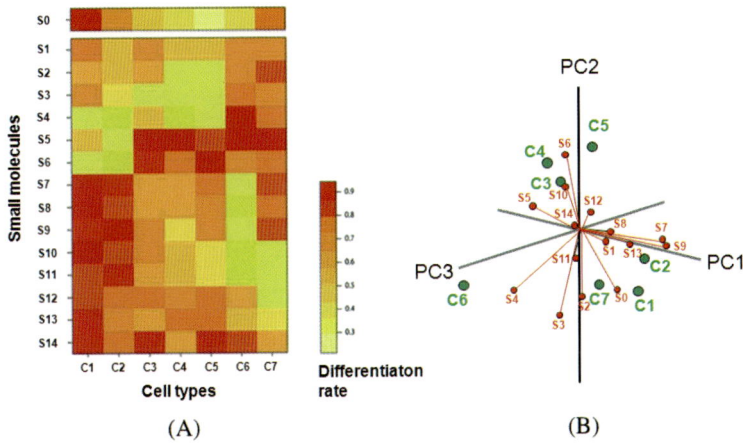

Fig. 2 Expression profile of target cell marker in MSCs treated with various small molecules. (A) Detection of relative expression level of cell markers by sandwich ELISA; (B) Differentiated effectiveness of small molecule by principal component analysis (PCA) method.

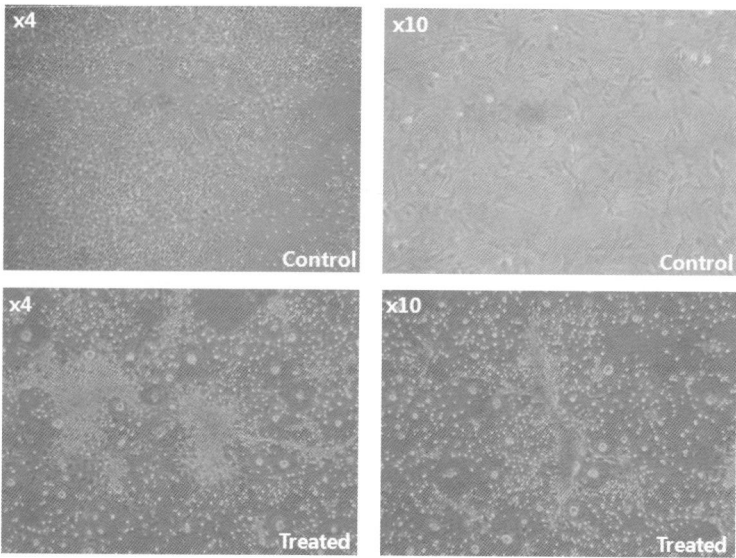

Fig. 3 Morphology of PKC activator treated MSCs (magnification ×4, 10).

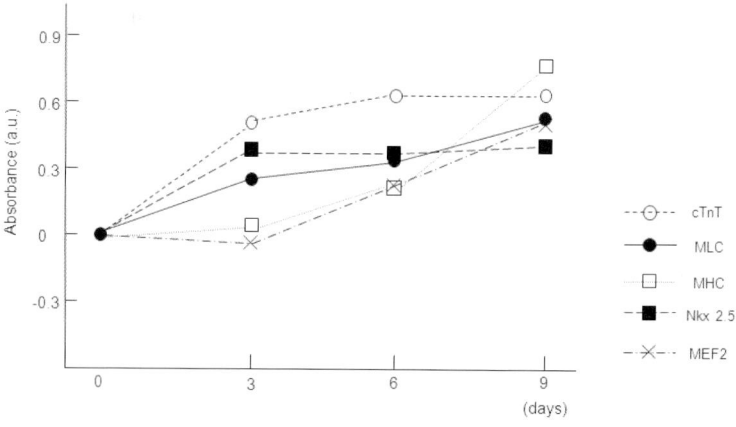

Fig. 4 Change of cardiac-specific marker in MSCs treated with PKC activator.

- Alpha-, beta-adrenergic receptor and muscarinic receptor were more expressed in cardiomyogenic cells compared with normal MSCs (Fig. 5).

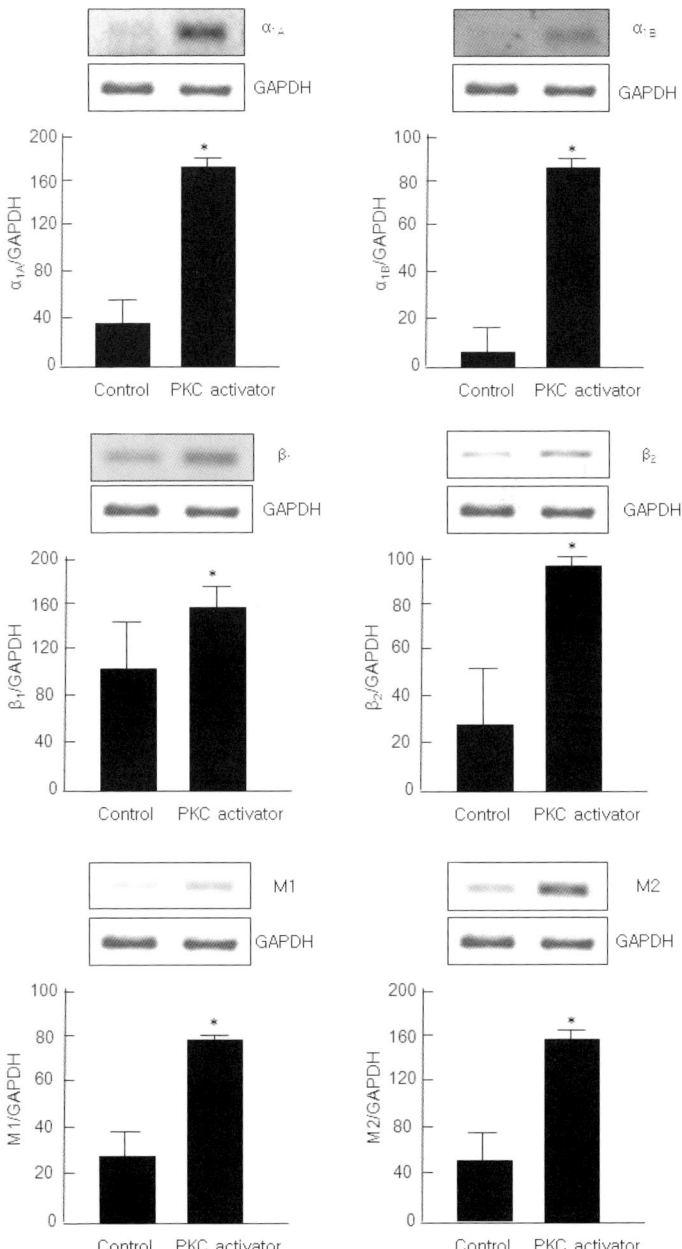

Fig. 5 Expression of alpha-, beta-adrenergic receptor and muscarinic receptor subtype in MSCs treated with PKC activator (*p < 0.01 vs. control).

- Effect of NE on phosphorylation of ERK1/2 was elevated in cardiomyogenic cells, time-dependently (Fig. 6).
- Expression of calcium handling-related protein (SERCA 2a and LTCC) was similar aspect to normal cardiomyocytes (Fig. 7).

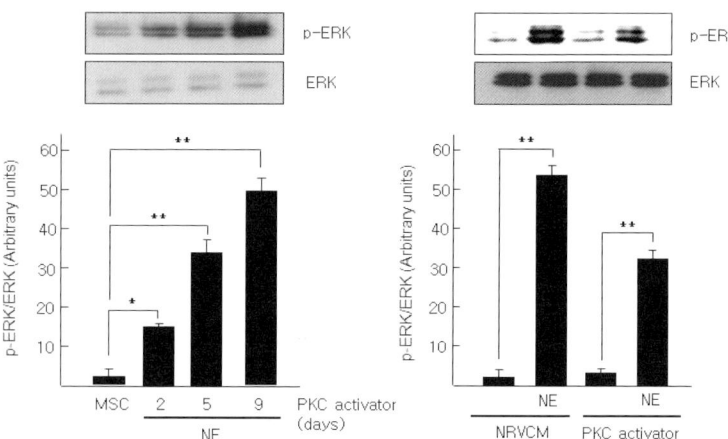

Fig. 6   The effect of NE on activation of ERK1/2 in MSCs treated with PKC activator (**p < 0.01 vs. each normal control).

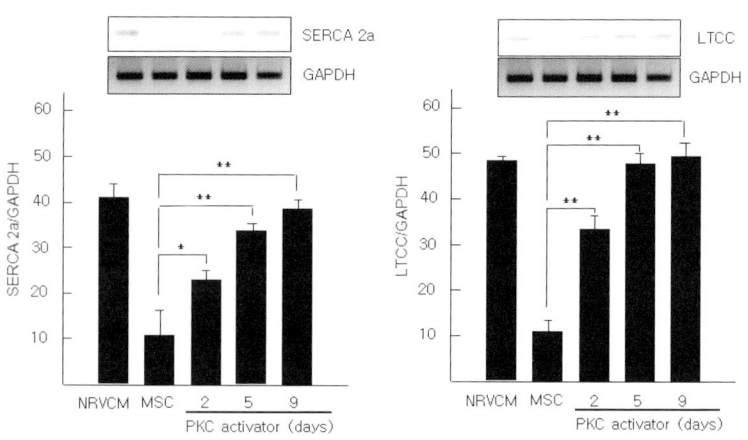

Fig. 7   The change of Ca^{2+}-related proteins in MSCs treated PKC activator (*,**p < 0.01 vs. MSC control).

Notes

- It is possible to change antibody for sandwich ELISA or immunocytochemistry, i.e. GATA4.
- In sandwich ELISA, incubation time point and antibody concentration can be various in researchers' method.
- PKC activator should be treated to MSCs for every 3 days.
- Remove the failure factors that affect the results in experiment (sandwich ELISA, cardiomyogenic cell of induction of time duration, etc).

M

Protocol for the Differentiation of BMSCs to a Smooth Muscle Cell for the Application of Engineering Small Diameter Blood Vessels

*Hyunhee Ahn, Young Min Ju and Sang Jin Lee**

*Wake Forest Institute for Regenerative Medicine, Wake Forest School of Medicine, Medical Center Boulevard, Winston-Salem, NC 27157, USA.

Background

- Cardiovascular disease, including coronary artery and peripheral vascular disease, is the leading cause of mortality in the United States (American Heart Association, 2012).
- The use of autologous vascular graft is considered to be the standard for small diameter (< 5 mm) blood vessels. However, more than 30% of patients are unable to use autologous veins due to additional invasive surgery and donor site necrosis.
- Although allografts and xenografts may offer long-term graft patency, their clinical utility is limited by the potential immunogenic response and pathogenic transfer.
- Synthetic grafts such as woven poly(ethylene terephthalate) (Dacron) and extended polytetrafluoroethylene (ePTFE) have been widely used for peripheral vascular reconstructions. However, these grafts tend to fail when they are applied to small-diameter (< 5 mm) vessels.
- Vascular tissue engineering attempts to create functional small diameter grafts by combining cells with a natural and/or synthetic scaffold material under suitable culture conditions, resulting in a tubular construct that can be used *in vivo*.
- An important consideration is the sourcing of vascular cells. Endothelial cells (ECs) and smooth muscle cells (SMCs) have functional significance in vessels. ECs are the key because they are anti-thrombogenic. SMCs contribute to contractility/tone and accelerate tissue maturation/formation, which provides mechanical stability. Further, the presence of SMCs in the implant may improve cellularization of the graft, which may in turn enhance resistance to infection, which is a common problem in prosthetic vascular grafts.
- Mature ECs and SMCs could be terminally differentiated cells with a low proliferative potential, and their capacity to expand to provide cells is limited.
- Adult stem cell-derived SMCs may be a promising alternative cell source. Recent research works showed that the ability of BMSCs to differentiate into SMCs was modulated by various growth factors, matrix proteins, and mechanical signals.

- Transforming growth factor β1 (TGF-β1) is the first member of the TGF-β superfamily that comprises bone morphogenic protein (BMP), antivin and subfamily of TGF-β. TGF-β1 acts as a major regulator in vasculogenesis in embryonic stage. It has been demonstrated that BMSCs could be differentiated into SMCs using TGF-β1 treatment as confirmed by expression of SMC specific markers such as α-SMA, SM-α22 as well as SM-MHC which involved in contractility.
- BMSCs differentiated into matured SMCs expressing SMC specific cytoskeletal proteins in the response to mechanical stimulation, especially compressive strain.
- Here, we present a method to differentiate human BMSCs into vascular SMCs using the combination of TGF-β1 treatment and pulsatile mechanical stimulation.

BMSC Isolation and Culture

- Human bone marrow is aspirated from upper posterior iliac crest from donor. Using density gradient centrifugal method, bone marrow is poured on top of Ficoll-Hypaque (1.077 g/mL, Sigma) solution and centrifuged at 445×g for 35 min.
- Ficoll-purified bone marrow mononuclear cells are plated into cell culture plates.
- Preparation of basal growth medium: Low glucose DMEM supplemented with 10% FBS and 1% of penicillin-streptomycin.

SMC Differentiation

- A stock solution for TGF-β1 (R&D Systems) is prepared by dissolving 2 μg of TGF-β1 in 1 mL of low glucose DMEM. 100 μl aliquot/tube is stored at −70°C.
- Preparation of differentiation medium: Low glucose DMEM supplemented with 5% FBS and 1% of penicillin-streptomycin and 5 ng/mL TGF-β1. Cells are cultured at 37°C in 5% CO_2, and culture medium is changed every 2 days.
- To optimize the concentration of TGF-β1, various concentrations of TGF-β1 (up to 10 ng/mL) were tested for differentiating hBMSCs into SMCs for 2 weeks of culture. Figure 1

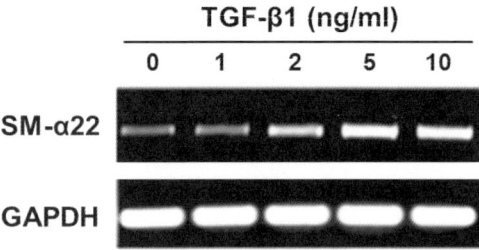

Fig. 1 RT-PCR analysis of SM-α22 gene expression in SMC differentiation with different concentrations of TGF-β1.

shows RT-PCR analysis of SM-α22 gene expression in SMC differentiation with different concentrations of TGF-β1 at 2 weeks after differentiation.

Immunocytochemistry for SMC Differentiation

- Primary antibodies: 1:500 dilution for α-smooth muscle actin (α-SMA), 1:100 dilution for smooth muscle-α22 (SM-α22), 1:200 dilution for smooth muscle-myosin heavy chain (SM-MHC), 1:100 dilution for calponin.
- Secondary antibodies: 1:200 dilution for Texas red conjugated anti-mouse IgG, anti-rabbit IgG, and anti-goat IgG (Invitrogen).
- Mounting medium to conserve expression of fluorescent: Vectashield Mounting Medium with 4'6-diamidine-2-phenylindole (DAPI) kit (Vector Laboratories Inc.).
- Fixation of the cells with 4% paraformaldehyde for 15 min.
- Permeabilization of the cells with 0.1% Triton-X100/PBS for 3 min at room temperature. Washing the cells 3 times with PBS for 3 min.
- Blocking of non-specific protein binding with serum-free protein blocker (DAKO) for 15 min.
- Primary antibodies diluted in antibody diluent solution (DAKO) and incubate 1 hr at room temperature in humidity chamber. Wash the cells 3 times with PBS for 3 min.
- Incubation of the cells with the fluorescent-conjugated secondary antibody for 45 min at RT. Wash the cells 3 times with PBS for 3 min.

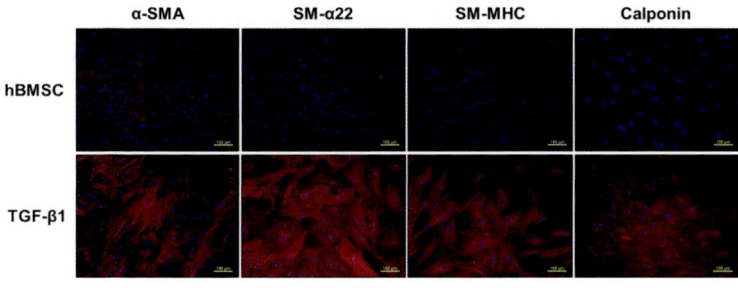

Fig. 2 Immunofluorescent images of expression of SMC specific markers in hBMSC after TGF-β1 treatment.

- Mount with fluorescent mounting medium and examine the cells.
- Figure 2 shows that immunofluorescent images of TGF-β1-treated BMSCs detected expression of the SMC specific markers.

RNA Extraction and Gene Expression Analysis

- Total RNA is isolated from hBMSCs using Trizol reagent (Invitrogen).
- cDNA is synthesized with 1 μg of total RNA and 1 μl of oligo-dT primers (0.4 μg/μL, Qiagene, CA, USA) and reverse transcription premix (Bioneer, Daejeon, Korea) as per manufacturer's instructions.
- To analyze SMC specific gene expression, a quantitative polymerase chain reaction (qPCR) can be performed. The qPCR condition is as follows: initial denaturation at 95°C for 10 min, then 50 cycles of amplification to denaturation at 94°C for 40 sec, annealing at 55°C for 40 sec, and extension at 72°C for 1 min, followed by a dissociation segment of 95°C for 1 min, 55°C for 30 sec and 95°C for 30 sec. The overall information of primer sequences is summarized in Table 1. The quantitative PCR reaction need to be performed in triplicate and the amount of the target gene is normalized by endogenous reference GAPDH. The comparative threshold cycle method is used according to the manufacturer's instructions for the analysis software used.

Table 1   Primers Used for qPCR.

Gene	Upper sequence	Lower sequence	Product size (bp)	Tm
GAPDH	ACTTCAACAGCGACACCCAC	TCCACCACCCTGTTGCTGTA	124	55°C
α-SMA	CGCCTCAGGAGATCAATGGC	TGCGTAGCCTCTCATTGTGC	111	55°C
SM-α22	GCTGGTGAACAGCCTGTACC	GCCTTCAGGAACTGAGCCAC	108	55°C
SM-MHC	GCAGCTCTTCAACCACACCA	CTCGATGAGCTCGATGCAGG	118	55°C

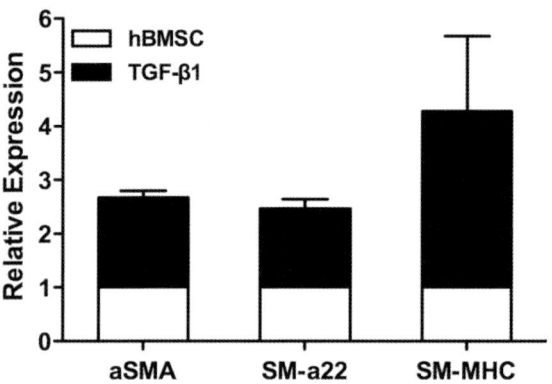

Fig. 3   SMC-specific gene expression (α-SMA, SM-α22, and SM-MHC) in hBMSCs after SMC differentiation induced by TGF-β1-treatment.

- As further analyzed of differentiation by real-time PCR quantitatively, Fig. 3 shows increased SMC-specific gene expression after treatment of TGF-β1. This indicates that TGF-β1 treatment could allow efficient differentiation of hBMSCs into SMCs.

Vascular Scaffold Fabrication (1, 2)

- Vascular scaffolds can be fabricated by electrospinning using a polymer blend of poly(ε-caprolactone) (PCL, iv=1.77 dL/g) and collagen type I derived from calf skin in 1,1,1,3,3,3-hexafluoro-2-propanol (HFIP).
- The electrospinning set-up includes a syringe pump, a high voltage supply, and a rotating mandrel to collect the fibers.

A positive voltage (5–25 kV) is applied to the polymer solution by the power supply. The PCL/collagen blend solution is delivered through an 18½ gauge blunt tip syringe needle at a constant flow rate of 1–10 mL/h using a syringe pump. The collecting mandrel is a 303 stainless steel rod (4.5 mm diameter). The distance between the syringe tip and the mandrel is 10–20 cm, and the rotation rate approximately 1000 rpm.

- Controllable variables in electrospinning include the solution concentration, flow rate, electric field strength, distance between tip and collector, needle tip design, and collector composition and geometry. These parameters can determine the fiber morphology, diameter, and alignment.
- Representative gross and SEM images showing the ultrastructure of the electrospun PCL/collagen scaffold are illustrated in Fig. 4. These electrospun vascular scaffolds possess excellent biomechanical properties and demonstrate a long-term stability under a continuous perfusion bioreactor system.

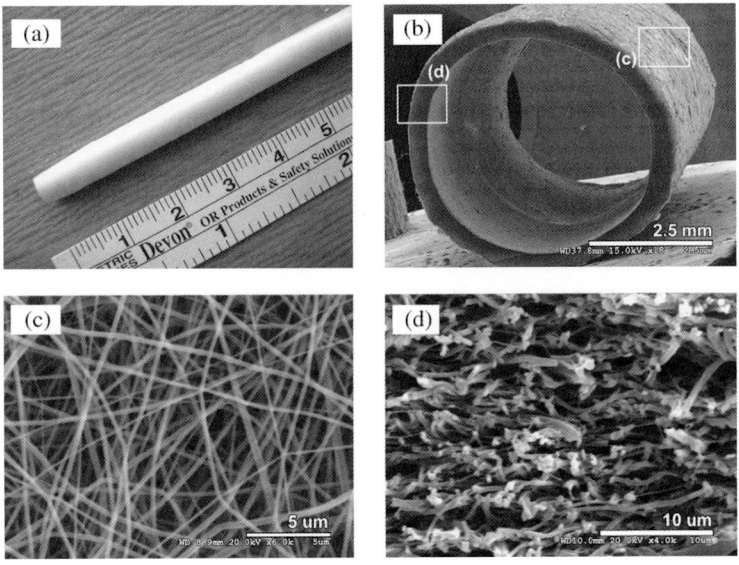

Fig. 4 (A) The gross appearance and SEM images of electrospun PCL/collagen scaffolds: (B) entire (×18), (C) surface (×6.0K), and (D) cross-sectional (×4.0K) morphologies (1).

Mechanical Stimulation Using a Pulsatile Bioreactor System

- Cell seeding: hBMSC-derived SMCs (cell density: 10^7 cells) are seeded on the outer layer of the electrospun PCL/collagen scaffold. After cell seeding, cell-seeded scaffold is incubated for 24 hr for cell adhesion. To further simulate blood flow, the cell-seeded tubular scaffolds are exposed to pulsatile flow conditions.
- Flow rates as reported above (0–1921 mL/min) are converted to shear stress values using the Hagen–Poiseuille equation, $\tau_{mean} = 4\mu Q/\pi R^3$, where Q is the volume flow rate, μ is the dynamic viscosity, and R is the lumen radius. This calculation yields values of τ_{mean} ranging from 0 to 63 dyne/cm^2.
- The bioreactor system developed for vascular applications allows for (a) seeding of vascular scaffolds, (b) generation and recording of physiologic flow, pressure, and stretch, (c) an external flow of media, (d) maintenance of gases and nutrients in the culture medium, and (e) maintenance of temperature and sterility.
- Cell-seeded vessel scaffold is mounted into a closed bioreactor, and the assembled bioreactor is connected to the system (Fig. 5A). Flow is initiated using a computer-operated gear pump (Ismatec MCP-Z Process, Glattbrugg, Switzerland) controlled by an Ismatec ProEdit program (V1.1.00). All

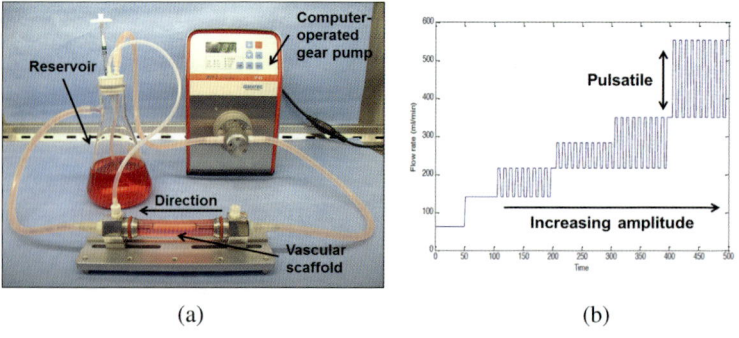

(a)   (b)

Fig. 5 Bioreactor system set-up for mechanical stimulation: (A) pulsatile perfusion bioreactor and (B) bioreactor protocol. The data acquisition and instrument control system delivers physiologic flow and pressure to the bioreactor which resides in an incubator.

components are contained within the incubator and kept at 37°C and 5% CO_2. Sterility is maintained throughout the pulsatile bioreactor process.

- Mechanical stimulation using the pulsatile bioreactor consists of graded increases in lumen flow rate and shear stress, with a transition from steady to pulsatile flow for at least 7 days, simulating arterial hemodynamic conditions (the vessel wall shear stress of 9.9 dyne/cm² in diastole and 13.2 dyne/cm² in systole). Supply a pulsatile flow waveform at a frequency of 60 cycles/min (Fig. 5B and Table 2).

- Figure 6 shows that pulsatile mechanical stimulation could promote differentiation of hBMSCs into SMCs on the electrospun PCL/collagen vascular scaffolds as confirmed by expression of α-SMA.

Table 2 Flow Rates for Pulsatile Bioreactor Set-Up.

Time (hr)	Flow rate (mL/min)	Status
0–50	50	Static
50–100	150	Static
100–200	150–250	Pulsatile
200–300	200–300	Pulsatile
300–400	200–350	Pulsatile
400–500	350–500	Pulsatile

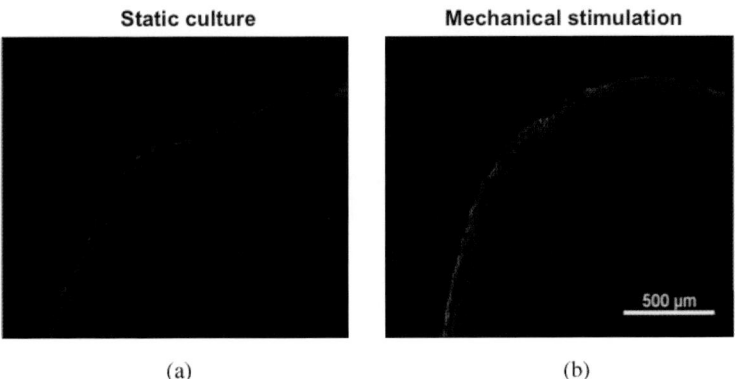

Static culture Mechanical stimulation

500 μm

(a) (b)

Fig. 6 Immunofluorescent images for α-SMA expression in hBMSC-derived SMC-seeded vascular scaffolds at 7 days of culture; (A) static culture and (B) mechanical stimulation using the pulsatile bioreactor.

Acknowledgments

This study was supported by the Telemedicine and Advanced Technology Research Center (TATRC) at the U.S. Army Medical Research and Material Command (USAMRMC) through award W81XWH-07-1-0718.

References

1. SJ Lee, J Liu, SH Oh, *et al.* (2008) Development of a composite vascular scaffolding system that withstands physiological vascular conditions. *Biomaterials* 29(19): 2891–2898.
2. YM Ju, JS Choi, A Atala, *et al.* (2010) Bilayered scaffold for engineering cellularized blood vessels. *Biomaterials* 31(15): 4313–4321.

N

Protocol of Schwann Cell Differentiation of BMSC by Direct Co-culture Method Using Insert System

Jeong Eun Song, Soon Hee Kim, Cho Min Kim and Gilson Khang*

*Dept of PolymerNano Sci & Tech., Dept of BIN Fusion Tech, and Polymer Fusion Research Center, Chonbuk National University, 567 Baekje-daero, Deokjin, Jeonju 561-756, Korea.

Background

- The autologous transplantation of Schwann cells (SCs) has become a routine clinical procedure for connecting nerve gaps in lesions of the peripheral nervous system (PNS).

- Axonal regeneration across nerve gaps in central nervous system (CNS) as well as in PNS is promoted by transplanting SCs alone or nerve conduits seeded with SCs.

- However, the culture of sufficient numbers of autologous SCs is time consuming and autologous SCs transplantation possesses possible alternation, including donor site morbidity, neuroma formation and infections.

- MSCs are multipotent stem cells that differentiate into cells of the mesodermal lineage by stimulation of stem cell using various reagents such as cytokines, growth factors and chemicals. In addition, MSCs show unusual plasticity to transdifferentiate into non-mesenchymal lineages such as astrocytes, myocardium, and myelinating cells of the peripheral nervous system and spinal cord when exposed to proper mitogens. Finally, BMSCs can be easily obtained by bone marrow suction and expanded over several subcultures maintaining their ability of differentiation.

- In this study, we will include the investigations into low the MSCs are able to give rise to SC-like cells when exposed to the environment of SC that possesses mitogens such as brain derived neurotrophic factor (BDNF) and glial growth factor (GGF) through co-culture of BMSCs and SCs of small quantity.

Culturing Methods of Schwann Cells

- SCs were harvested and purified from neonatal rat sciatic nerve according to a previously developed Morrissey's method (Fig. 1).

- Aseptically remove sciatic nerves from neonatal rats and rinse them with PBS.

- Dissect with microscissors the epineurium and connective tissue on petri-dish supplemented with DMEM/F12 medium.

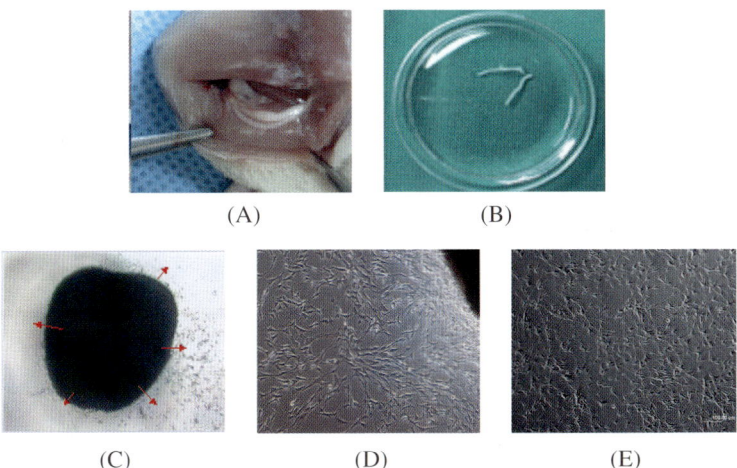

Fig. 1 The processing of SCs isolation. (A) Existing sciatic nerve in rat thigh. (B) Harvested sciatic nerve before chopping. (C) Fibroblast outgrowth from fragments of sciatic nerve (×40). (D) Fibroblast outgrowth from fragments of sciatic nerve (×100). (E) SCs purified after 7th tissue transfer (×100).

- Chop sciatic nerves into the length of 1–2 mm and culture fragments of 5–7 in non-treated well plate (diameter 3.5 cm) with DMEM/F12 medium supplemented with 10% FBS, 1% antibiotics (100 unit/mL penicillin and 100 µg/mL streptomycin), 2 µM forskolin and 20 µg/mL bovine pituitary extract for 7 days.
- Transfer the fragments of nerve into new plate and culture them for 7 days in order to exclude fibroblast outgrowth from nerves. Repeat this transfer process 7 times.
- Treat with 0.1% collagenase and 0.1% trypsin (1:1) and put them for 30 min at 37°C in 7th transfer of tissue fragments.
- Strain out digested tissue using strainer (100 µm) and rinse filtered cells.
- Plate the cells at a density of 1×10^5 cells/75cm^2 on poly-L-lysine-coated (100 µg/mL) tissue culture flask with DMEM/F12 medium containing 10% FBS, 1% antibiotics (100 unit/mL penicillin and 100 µg/mL streptomycin), 2µM forskolin and 20 µg/mL bovine pituitary extract.
- Use the cells of 1–4 passages.

SCs Characterization

- Anti-S100, GFAP, p75 (LNGF-R), and Gal C+ as SCs marker and anti-Thy-1 as fibroblast marker confirmation by immunocytochemistry (ICC) or immunofluorescence (IF).

Co-culture with BMSCs and SCs

- Put poly(L-lysine) coated Millicell culture plate inserts on the well.
- Seed SCs onto the surface of Millicell culture plate inserts at a density of 1×10^4 cells/filter.
- Culture BMSCs combined with SCs with DMEM containing 10% FBS and 1% antibiotics (100 unit/mL penicillin and 100 µg/mL streptomycin).
- Remove medium from co-culture system next day and add fresh medium.
- Maintain culture for up to 3 weeks.

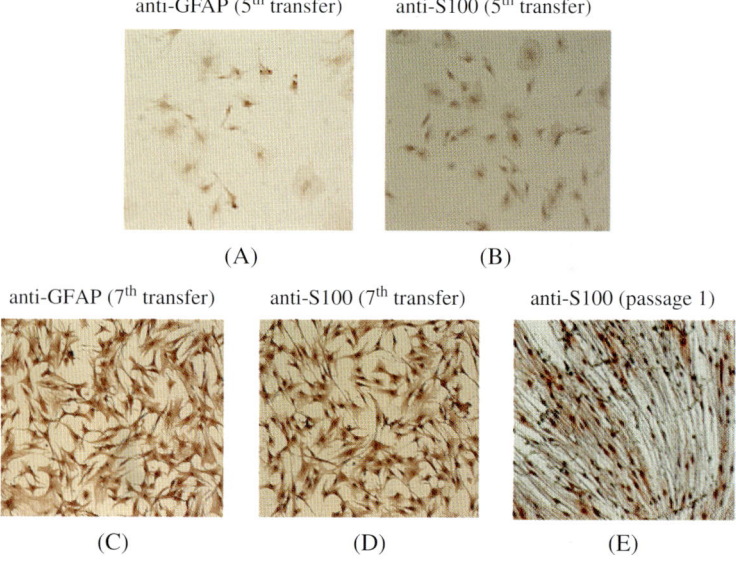

Fig. 2 Analysis of purification in cultured SCs.

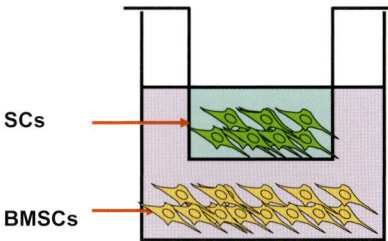

Fig. 3 Diagram of indirect co-culture system using BMSC and SCs.

Analysis for SCs Induction of BMSCs

- Anti-S100, p75(LNGF-R), GFAP, AN2 and Gal C+ as SCs marker confirmation by ICC or IF.
- Detection of S100, p75, GFAP, CD104 and Krox-20 mRNA for SCs marker using RT-PCR.

Requirements

DMEM (low glucose), DMEM and Ham's F-12, forskolin, BPE, antibiotics (100 unit/mL penicillin and 100 μg/mL streptomycin), PBS, trypsin-EDTA, FBS, Collagenase I, 6-well plate, poly(L-lysine), single-well cell culture inserts

Characterization

- BMSCs cultured without SCs show no DAB expression when immunostained for GFAP, S100 and P75 (Figs. 4–6A).
- GFAP, S100 and P75 exhibit strong immunopositivity in BMSCs cultured with SCs (Figs. 4–6B).
- The level of expression of three markers in co-culture group is not significantly different to that observed in SCs (Figs. 4–6C).
- BMSCs cultured without SCs show weakly S100 mRNA (Fig. 7A).
- BMSCs cultured with SCs show strongly S100 mRNA (Fig. 7B).
- The level of S100 mRNA expression in co-culture group is not different to that observed in SCs (Fig. 7C).

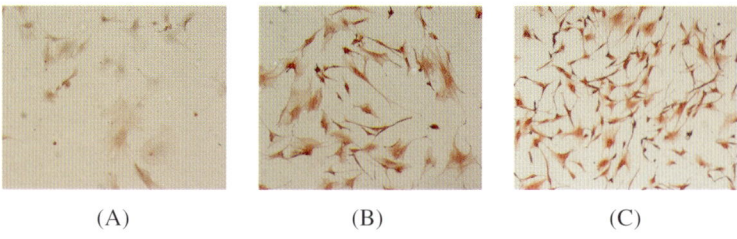

(A) (B) (C)

Fig. 4 ICC for anti-GFAP at day 21 with co-culture, (A) BMSCs, (B) BMSCs co-cultured with SCs, (C) SCs (magnification ×100) [2].

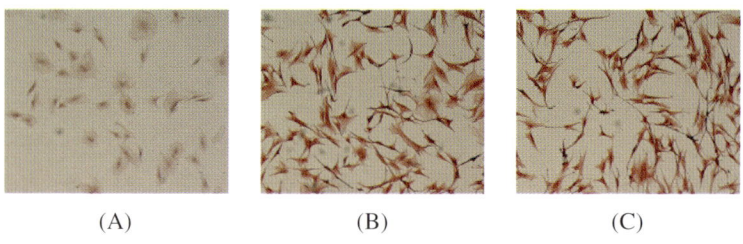

(A) (B) (C)

Fig. 5 ICC for anti-S100 at day 21 with co-culture, (A) BMSCs, (B) BMSCs co-cultured with SCs, (C) SCs (magnification ×100) [1].

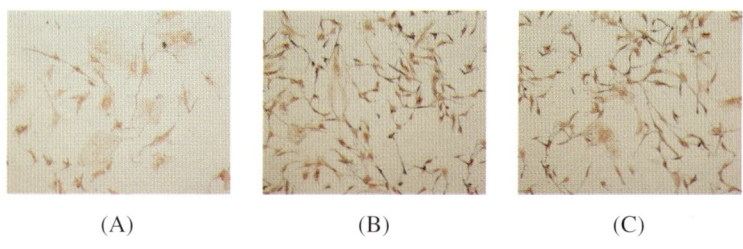

(A) (B) (C)

Fig. 6 ICC for anti-P75 at day 21 co-culture, (A) BMSCs, (B) BMSCs co-cultured with SCs, (C) SCs (magnification × 100).

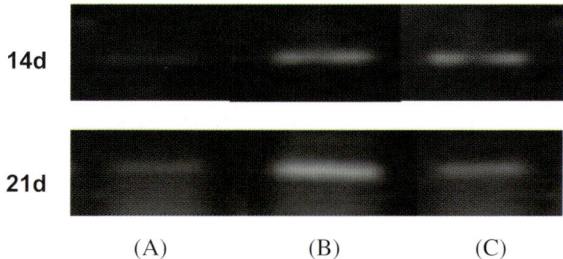

(A) (B) (C)

Fig. 7 Expression of S100 mRNA levels using RT-PCR. (A) BMSCs, (B) BMSCs co-cultured with SCs, (C) SCs.

Notes

- It is possible to add glial growth factor to enhance induction into SCs of BMSCs.
- We suggest to evaluate mRNA for MSC marker (e.g. BMPR-1A) using RT-PCR post differentiation into SCs.

Acknowledgments

This research was supported by WCU (R31-20029, KMEST), Bio-industry Technology Development Program (112007-05-1-SB010, MKFAFF) and Bio & Medical Technology Development Program (2012M3A9C6050204, KMEST).

References

1. CM Kim, SM Kim, SH Kim, *et al.* (2007) Effect of Schwann cell on differentiation of bone marrow stromal cells. *Tiss Eng Regen Med* **4**(1): 60–66.
2. CM Kim, SH Kim, Y Song, *et al.* (2009) Co-cultuer of schwann cell and bone marrow stromal cells on differentiation and proliferation of bone marrow stromal cells. *Tiss Eng Regen Med* **6**(4–11): 882–887.

O

Protocol of Neurogenesis of BMSC Using β-Mercaptoethanol Released System from β-Mercaptoethanol-Loaded PLGA Film

Jeong Eun Song, Eun Young Kim, Hyeon Yoon, Dongwon Lee and Gilson Khang*

*Dept of BIN Fusion Tech, Polymer Fusion Res Center & Dept of PolymerNanoSci Tech, Chonbuk National Univ, 567 Baekje-daero, Deojin, Jeonju 561-756 Korea.

Background

- Stem cells have received much attention as a treatment for cardiovascular, neural, and hereditary diseases which were considered incurable diseases in the past. Due to their potential to integrate into the host tissue, to replace lost cells, and to repair the injured tissues, a number of researchers have studied their potential in regenerative medicine.

- BMSCs, a type of adult stem cell, have the potential to differentiate into other cells, such as that of fat, bone, and cartilage. Recently, neuronal differentiation of BMSCs has also been reported.

- Sustained-release scaffolds, which release bioactive factors slowly, are important in the field of tissue engineering because bioactive factors required for cell differentiation can be degraded easily due to their short half-life in culture medium.

- We focused our attention on the poly(L-lactide-*co*-glycolide) (PLGA)/β-mercaptoethanol (BME) hybrid polymeric scaffold, which can release BME slowly to attached cells, and investigated whether BMSCs would differentiate into neural cells when cultured in PLGA/BME hybrid polymeric films.

Fabrication of PLGA/BME Film

- A BME-impregnated PLGA film was prepared by dissolving PLGA 5% (v/v) in dichloromethane.

- BME (0, 200, 400 and 600 μM of PLGA) was then thoroughly dispersed.

- The PLGA/BME solution was cast into a glass petri dish (50 mm in diameter).

- The solvent was evaporated at room temperature, with the film being produced.

- The PLGA/BME film was removed gently from the mold using forceps and dried under a vacuum at room temperature for 3 days.

- Preparation of PLGA films that contain various concentrations of BME is shown (Fig. 1A).

- Colorless and transparent circular PLGA/BME hybrid films were obtained (Fig. 1B).

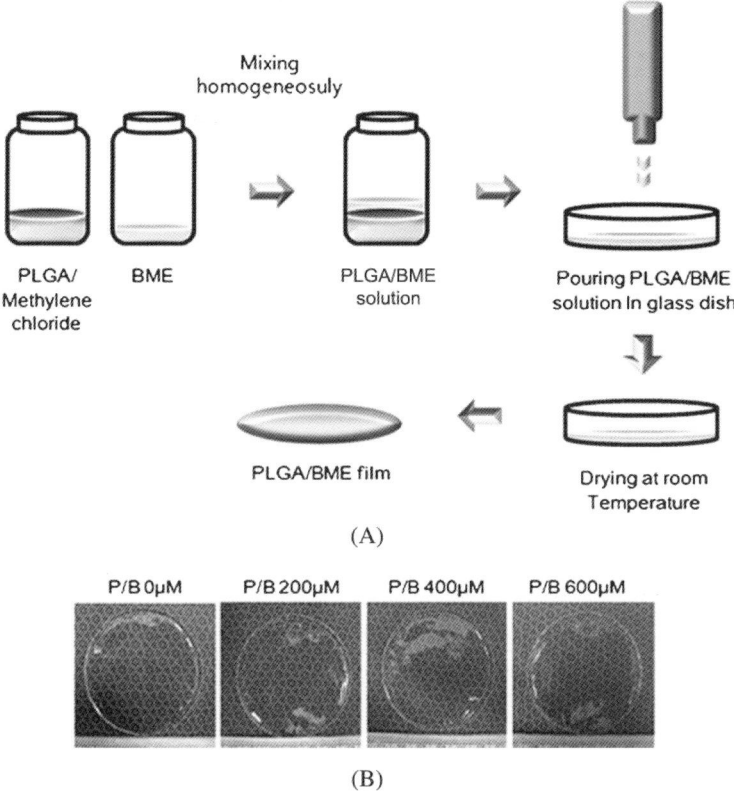

Fig. 1 Schematic diagram illustrating the fabrication process of PLGA/BME film.[1]

Analysis for Neurogenesis *In Vitro* and *In Vivo*

- Immunohistochemistry to verify the expression of specific protein in BMSCs.
- Water absorption of PLGA/BME hybrid films to confirm the effect of BME on the films.
- Metabolic activity of BMSCs on the hybrid films depend on the concentration of BME.
- RT-PCR to confirm whether BMSCs expressed neuronal cell markers on the PLGA/BME films.
- SEM to observe the morphology of BMSCs on PLGA/BME films.

Requirements

A medium: DMEM (low glucose) supplemented with 10% FBS and 0 µM of BME as a control, DMEM supplemented with 10% FBS and 200 µM, 400 µM, 1 mM, 5 mM and 10 mM of BME (Table 1A).

B medium: DMEM with 20% DMSO, 25 mM of potassium chloride, 2 mM valporic acid, 10 µM forskolin, 5 µg/mL insulin, and 1 µM hydrocortisone for 15 hr (Table 1B).

Characterization

- BME plays an important role in both differentiating the cells and maintaining the cells in a differentiated state (Fig. 2).
- The medium with appropriate concentrations of BME presented a higher cell density and certain morphology (Fig. 3).

Table 1   Composition of cell culture media. A; neuronal differentiation of BMSCs on Well. B; neuronal differentiation of BMSCs on PLGA/BME film.

A

Differentiation	Medium	Supplementation
Cell adhesion	DMEM	10% FBS, 1% PS
Induction	DMEM	10% FBS, 100 µM BME
Pre-induction	DMEM	20% DMSO, 10% FBS, 10 ng/mLb FGF
Neuronal differentiation	DMEM	10% FBS, 200 µM, 400 µM, 1 mM, 5 mM, 10 mM BME

B

Differentiation	Medium	Supplementation
Cell adhesion	DMEM	10% FBS, 1% PS
Pre-induction	DMEM	10% FBS, 10 ng/mLb FGF
Neuronal differentiation	DMEM	20% DMSO, 10% FBS
Long-term neuronal differentiation	DMEM	20% DMSO, 25 mM KCl, 2 mM valporic acid, 10 µM forskolin, 1 µM hydrodortisone, 5 µg/mL insulin

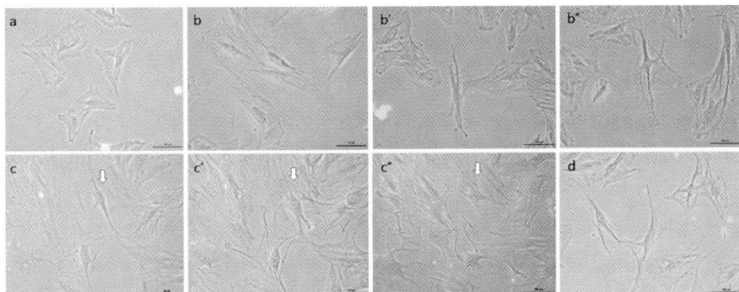

Fig. 2 Observation of morphological changes of BMSCs by inverted microscopic pictures. The typical morphology of BMSCs (a) Morphological changes of BMSCs after incubation.[1]

- The influence of BME on the differentiation of BMSCs into neural-like cells depends on the concentration of BME in the medium, and it is important to include the appropriate concentration of BME in PLGA/BME hybrid films in order to differentiate BMSCs into neural-like cells with reduced apoptosis (Fig. 4).

- Through results of the comparison of contact angle between PLGA films and PLGA/BME hybrid films, we found that PLGA/BME hybrid film containing 200 μM BME has an excellent hydrophilic profile (Fig. 5).

- We observed inverted microscopic pictures of neuronal differentiation of BMSCs on PLGA/BME film and confirmed that the medium that we used could differentiate BMSCs into neural-like cells in both tissue culture plates and PLGA/BME hybrid films (Fig. 6).

- The similar cell viabilities were observed in all experimental films, thus indicating that our PLGA/BME hybrid films can be used for long-term culture and can increase the cell proliferation rate (Fig. 7).

- The results of NF analysis indicate that the addition of certain amounts of BME is required to induce BMSCs into neural-like cells. We believe that BME has more influence on PLGA/BME films than PLGA film through the continuous release of BME (Fig. 8).

- The uncertain morphology and low cell density of BMSCs cultured with high concentrations of BME show the high toxicity by high concentration of BME (Fig. 9).

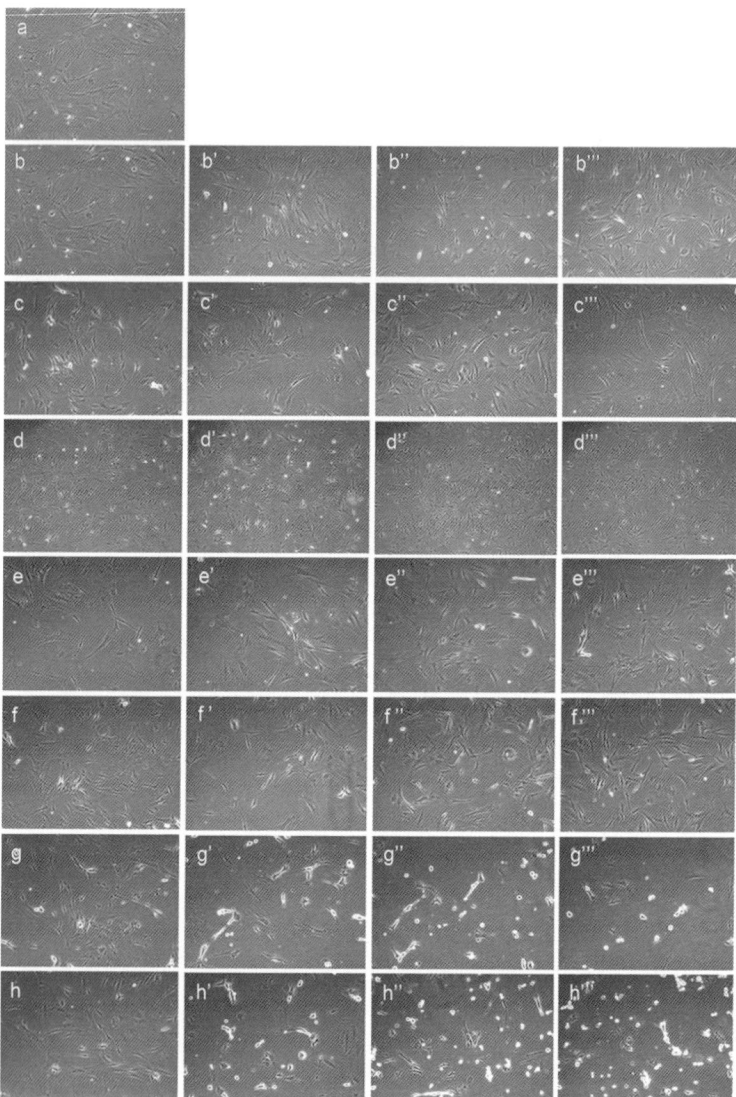

Fig. 3 Inverted microscope pictures of BMSCs in neural differentiation medium: (a) cell adhesion, (b–b'''); pre-induction and (c–h'''); neuronal differentiation (c–c'''); BME 0 μM, (d–d'''); BME 200 μM, (e–e'''); BME 400 μM, (f–f'''); BME 1 mM, (g–g'''); BME 5 mM, (h–h'''); BME 10 mM). Scale bar = 100 μm.[1]

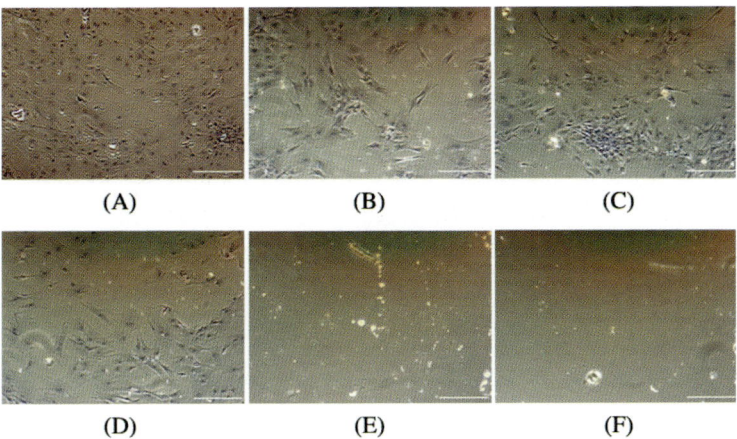

Fig. 4 Inverted microscopic pictures of cell morphology according to immunohistochemical staining for NF (a) BME 0 μM, (b) BME 200 μM, (c) BME 400 μM, (d) BME 1 mM, (e) BME 5 mM, (f) BME 10 mM) Scale bar = 100 μm.

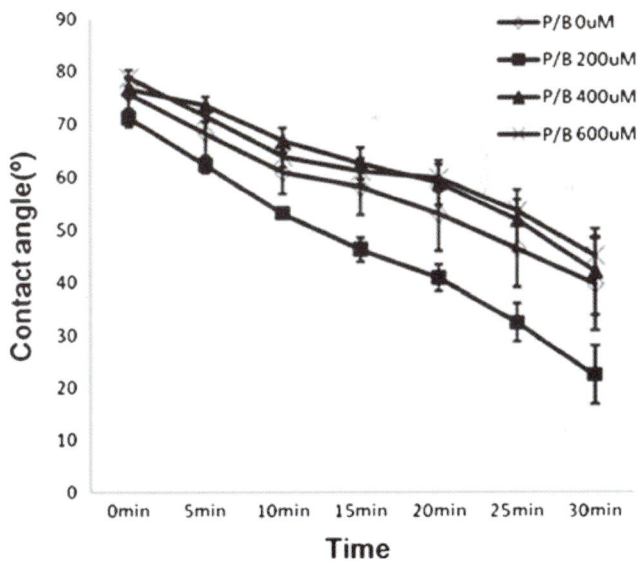

Fig. 5 Water-uptake experiments using PLGA/BME (0, 200, 400 and 600 μM) film.[1]

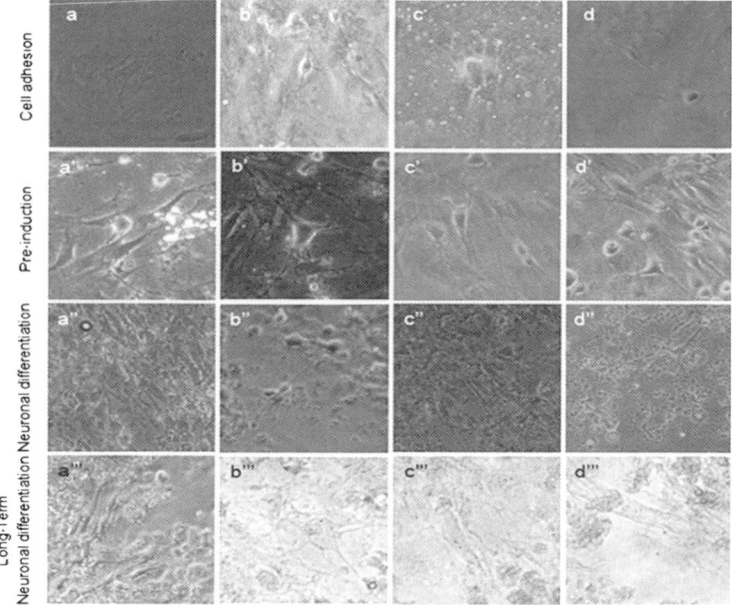

Fig. 6 Inverted microscopic pictures of neuronal differentiation of BMSCs on PLGA/BME film. (a–a''') 0 μM, (b–b''') 200 μM, (c–c''') 400 μM, (d–d''') 600 μM; and (a–d'') magnification ×200, Scale bar = 100 μm, (a'''-d'''); magnification ×400. Scale bar = 50 μm.

Notes

- To add controlled amount of BME will promote BMSCs to differentiate into neural-like cells without cell shrinkage or apoptosis.
- It was found that only PLGA/BME hybrid films containing 200 μM BME exhibited a higher hydrophilicity than PLGA films, demonstrated that it has an excellent hydrophilic profile.
- PLGA/BME hybrid films can have many applications, not only in tissue regeneration but also for neuralized implants using BMSCs.

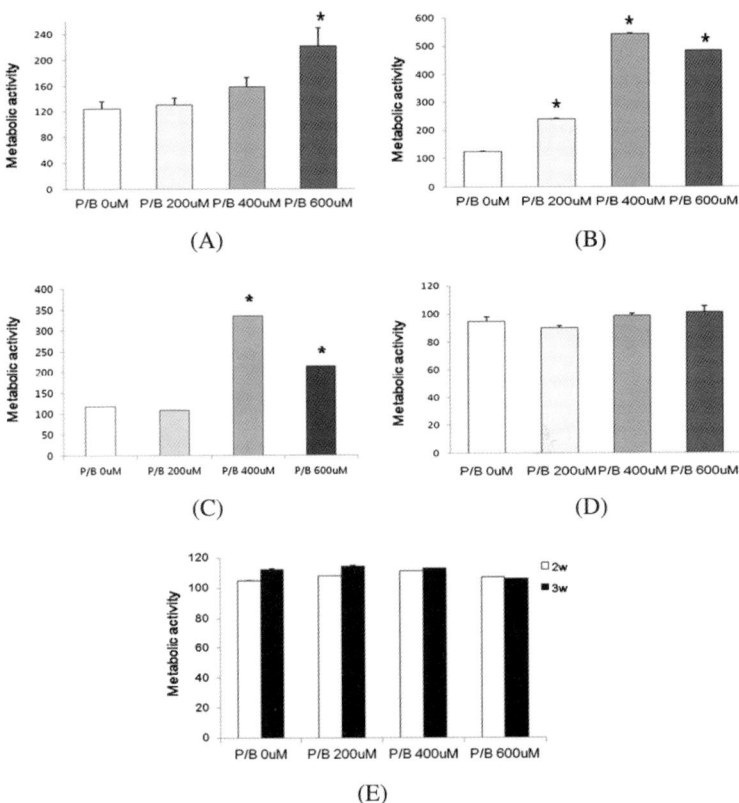

Fig. 7 Metabolic activity of BMSCs in PLGA/BME film analyzed by WST assay: (a) cell adhesion medium for 4 days, (b) pre-induction medium for 1 day, (c) neuronal differentiation medium for 5 hr, (d) long-term neuronal differentiation medium for 15 hr, and (e) long-term neuronal differentiation medium for 2 and 3 weeks (* $p < 0.05$ vs. P/B 0 μM).

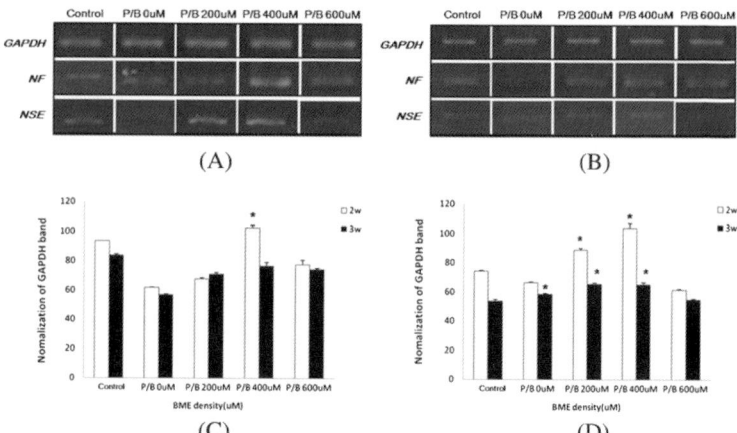

Fig. 8 The results of agarose gel electrophoresis: Effect of varying BME density on neuronal gene expression in BMSC markers 2 (a) and 3 weeks (b) expression of related NF (c) and NSE (d) genes by BMSCs cultured on the PLGA/BME film for 2 and 3 weeks. Levels, quantified using RT-PCR, are normalized to the housekeeping gene, GAPDH ($* $ $p < 0.05$ vs. control).[1]

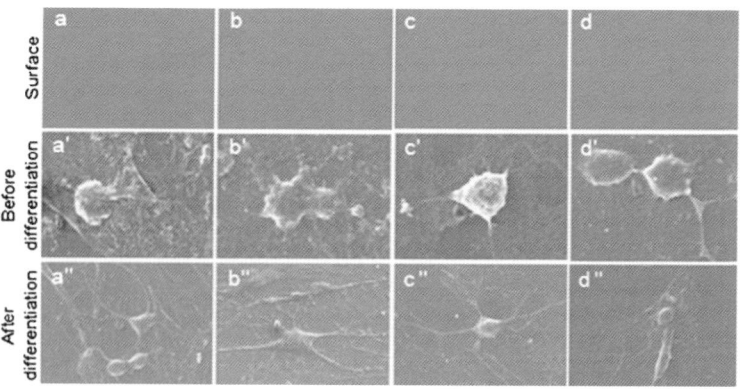

Fig. 9 SEM microphotographs of BMSC attachment pattern and the proliferative responsiveness on PLGA/BME film surfaces (a–d), before differentiation (a'–d') and after differentiation (a''–d''): (a–a''); P/B 0 μm, (b–b''); P/B 200 μm, (c–c''); P/B 400 μm, (d–d''), P/B 600 μm and (a'–d'); magnification ×20 k, scale bar = 20 μm, (a''–d''); magnification ×1.0 k, scale bar = 50 μm.[1]

Acknowledgments

This research was supported by WCU (R31-20029, KMEST), Bio-industry Technology Development Program (112007-05-1-SB010, MKFAFF) and Bio & Medical Technology Development Program (2012M3A9C6050204, KMEST).

Reference

1. G Khang, HL Kim, M Hong, D Lee. (2012) Neurogenesis of bone marrow-derived mesenchymal stem cells onto β-mercaptoethanol-loaded PLGA film. *Cell Tissue Res* **347**: 713–724.

P

Protocol of Neural Differentiation from BMSCs Using bFGF and Laminin-Coating Plate

Byung Hyune Choi, Jin-Mo Kim and So Ra Park

Division of Biomedical and Bioengineering Sciences, Inha University College of Medicine, Incheon 400-712, Korea.

Background

- Adult BMSCs are a valuable source of cell therapy for human diseases and stem cell research. They can be easily obtained, expand rapidly and differentiate into various cell types *in vitro*.

- MSCs can basically differentiate into mesenchymal lineages such as osteoblasts, chondroblasts, and adipocytes. In addition, many studies also demonstrated that MSCs could differentiate into various non-mesenchymal tissues under appropriate experimental conditions *in vitro* and *in vivo*, such as hepatocytes, cardiomyocytes, lung alveolar epithelium, and even neuron and glia.

- Many protocols to differentiate MSCs into neural lineage have been developed using various growth factors and small chemicals such as nerve growth factor (NGF), brain-derived neurotrophic factor (BDNF), retinoic acid (RA) and β-mercaptoethanol. There are also neural differentiation media for MSCs and neural progenitor cells (NPCs) commercially available on the market. However, no specified protocol highly efficient for neural differentiation of MSCs has been established yet.

- It has also been reported that the microenvironment of MSCs during the differentiation period could also affect neural differentiation efficiency of MSCs. In particular, the effect of cell adhesion molecules such as collagen, laminin and fibronectin are being widely studied in monolayer or 3-D culture.

- We used basic fibroblast growth factor (bFGF) and laminin as a cell adhesion substrates for neural differentiation of rat MSCs. The effect of laminin-coating plate was compared with those of normal cell culture plate and poly(L-lysine) (PLL)-coating plate.

Isolation and Culture Expansion of Rat MSCs

- Isolate mononuclear cells (MNCs) from the femurs and tibias of young Sprague-Dawley rats (100 g).

- Wash the MNCs with PBS and suspend in alpha-MEM containing 10% FBS, 100 U/mL penicillin and 100 µg/mL

Isolated BMNCs (P0)	Remove the non-adherent cells (P0)	P1

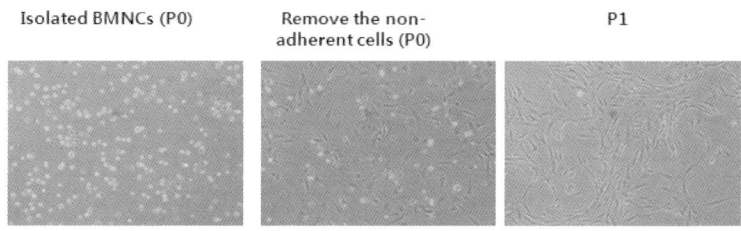

Fig. 1 Morphology of rMSCs during the primary culture (P: passage, magnification ×100).

streptomycin. They were cultured at a density of 10^4–10^5 cell/cm^2 in a humidified atmosphere under 5% CO_2 at 37°C.

- The non-adherent cells were removed after 1 week of culture and adherent cells were maintained until 90% confluence, when cells were harvested by trypsinization (0.05% trypsin-EDTA) and then replated at 1/4 dilution ratio.
- The culture medium was changed every 3–4 days during the expansion period and rat MSCs of early passages (P2–P4) were used for the differentiation experiments.
- Isolated MSCs showed fibroblast-like morphology (Fig. 1).

Characterization of BMSCs

- Analyze properties of rat MSCs at passage 2 by flow cytometry using known cell surface markers for MSCs (CD44, CD105, CD90) (Fig. 2). Whereas BMSCs were lacking CD45- and CD34- as hematopoietic stem cell markers (data not shown).
- Examine the capacity of the BMSCs to differentiate in the adipogenic, osteogenic and chondrogenic lineages (Fig. 3).

Preparation of Laminin- or PLL-Coating Plate

- Dilute laminin and PLL in α-MEM without FBS at 20 μg/mL and 10 μg/mL, respectively.
- Add enough volume of diluted laminin or PLL solution to cover the tissue culture plate (use 3 mL for 6 cm plate and 6.5 mL for 10 cm plate).

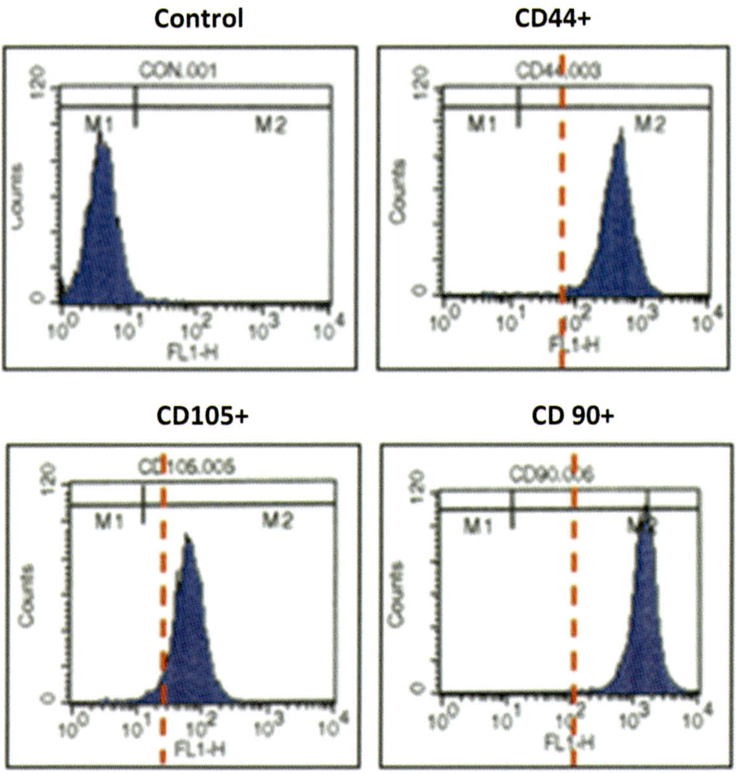

Control
CD44+
CD105+
CD 90+
CON.001
M1
M2
Counts
FL1-H

Fig. 2 Surface marker gene expression of BMSC.

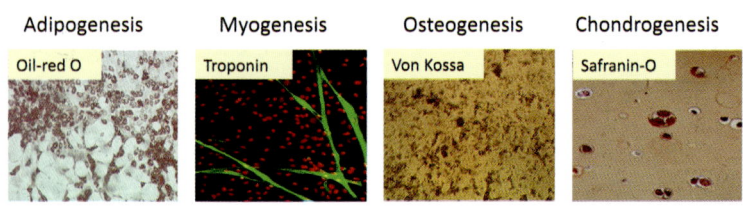

Adipogenesis
Myogenesis
Osteogenesis
Chondrogenesis
Oil-red O
Troponin
Von Kossa
Safranin-O

Fig. 3 Differentiation potential of rat MSCs into mesenchymal lineages.

- Incubate the plates containing laminin or PLL solution in a humidified atmosphere under 5% CO_2 at 37°C for at least 4 hr.
- Aspirate the laminin or PLL solution from the coated plate and rinse the plate once with 1X PBS or culture medium.

- The laminin-coating plates can be stored at −20°C for 6–8 months. The plates should be wrapped with a foil or a plastic wrap for long-term storage.

Neural Differentiation of rMSCs

- Seed rMSCs at 1×10^5 cells/mL in the culture plate containing expansion medium (α-MEM + 10% FBS) at 1 day before neural differentiation.
- The next day, remove the expansion medium by aspiration and wash the cells twice with PBS.
- Incubate cells in serum-free neural differentiation medium (α-MEM containing B27, N2 (Gibco) and 10 ng/mL FGF-2) in a humidified atmosphere under 5% CO_2 at 37°C for 2 days.
- After 2 days, add 100 ng/mL NGF, 10 ng/mL EGF, 100 ng/mL BDNF and 10 nM RA all at final concentrations to each culture medium.
- Further incubate cells for 2 weeks with the culture medium replaced every 3–4 days. The final neural differentiation medium contains all growth factors and compounds used.

Analysis of Neural Differentiation of rMSCs

- Observe the neural morphorolgy.
- Immunostaining for the expression of neural marker genes.
- RT-PCR for the expression of neural marker genes.
- Neural marker genes include nestin, sox2, glial fibrillary acidic protein (GFAP), b III-tubulin, and neurofilament-M (NF-M), etc.

Requirements

Young Sparague-Dawley rats (100 g), α-MEM, antibiotics (100 U/mL penicillin and 100 μg/mL streptomycin), PBS, trypsin-EDTA, FBS, B27 and N2 supplements, bFGF, NGF, EGF, BDNF, RA, antibodies, PCR primers and cell culture wares.

Characterization

- The proliferation of rat MSCs was significantly increased (at passage 2) when cells were cultured on laminin-coating plates in expansion medium compared to those on normal culture plate and PLL-coating plate (Fig. 4).
- Under the neural differentiation condition, the laminin-coating plate showed no clear difference from the normal culture plate or PLL-coating plate in the nestin (early marker) expression, but showed significant increase in the expression of GFAP, NF-M and b III-tubulin (late markers) (Fig. 5). This result suggests that laminin-coating might have played a key role in the late step of neural differentiation not in the early commitment of rat MSCs into neural progenitor state.
- During the neural differentiation of rat MSCs on laminin-coating plate, treatment of bFGF for 2 days significantly

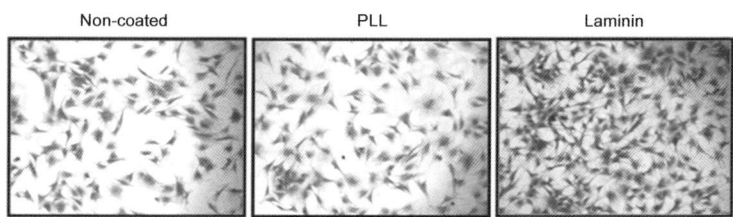

Fig. 4 The effect of laminin in the proliferation of rMSCs.

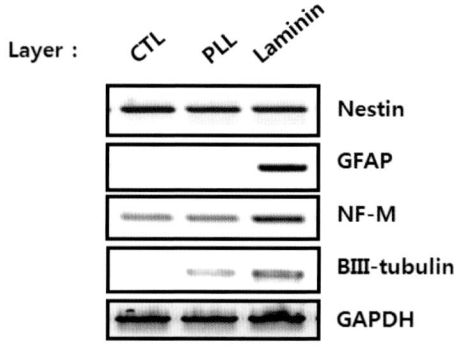

Fig. 5 The effect of laminin on the differentiation of rMSCs.

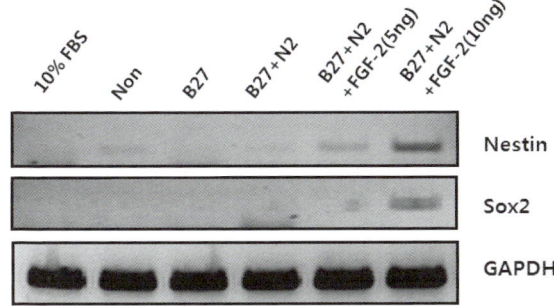

Fig. 6 The effect of FGF-2 on the neural commitment of rMSCs.

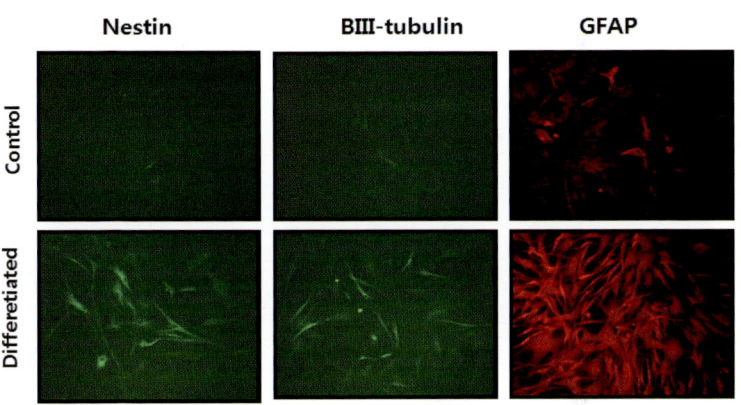

Fig. 7 The expression of neural marker genes.

increased expression of nestin and sox2, the NPCs markers in the RT-PCR analysis (Fig. 6). This result showed that bFGF might be essential in the early commitment of rat MSCs into NPCs state.

- The expression of nestin, BIII-tubulin, and GFAP was significantly induced then, when additional factors (NGF, EGF, BDNF and RA) were added but not in the control group in the immunocytochemical analysis (Fig. 7).

- Taken together, our results suggest that both culture microenvironment like laminin coating and combination of growth factors and chemicals are necessary to induce efficient differentiation of rat MSCs to the neural lineage.

References

1. P Tropel, N Platet, JC Platel, *et al.* (2007) Functional neuronal differentiation of bone marrow-derived mesenchymal stem cells. *Stem Cells* **25**(2): 543.
2. Z Lei, L Yongda, M Jun, *et al.* (2007) Culture and neural differentiation of rat bone marrow mesenchymal stem cells *in vitro. Cell Biol Int* **31**(9): 916–923.
3. A Hermann, S Liebau, R Gastl, *et al.* (2006) Comparative analysis of neuroectodermal differentiation capacity of human bone marrow stromal cells using various conversion protocols. *J Neurosci Res* **83**(8):1502–1514.
4. P Bossolasco, L Cova, C Calzarossa, *et al.* (2005) Neuro-glial differentiation of human bone marrow stem cells *in vitro. Exp Neurol* **193**(2): 312–325.

Q

Protocol of Differentiation of Retinal Pigment Epithelial-like Cells from BMSC Using Co-culture Method

Su Ji Kang*, Eun Young Kim*, Hyeon Yoon*, Chun-Ki Joo† and Gilson Khang*,‡

---

* Dept of BIN Fusion Tech, Polymer Fusion Res Center & Dept of Polymer Nano Sci Tech, Chonbuk National Univ, 567 Baekje-daero, Deokjin, Jeonju 561-756, Korea.

† Department of Ophthalmology and Visual Science, College of Medicine, The Catholic University of Korea, Gangnam St. Mary Hospital, Korea, 505 Banpo-dong, Seocho-gu, Seoul 137-701.

Background

- Retinal pigment epithelium (RPE) plays a key role in the maintenance of normal functions and health of the neural retina. Important metabolic functions of RPE cells also include active transport of ions, water and vitamin A, and phagocytosis of the photoreceptor outer segment.
- Conditions of retinal degeneration including retinitis pigmentosa (RP) and age-related macular degeneration (AMD) affect over a million people, where they comprise the leading cause of irreversible visual disability.
- BMSCs were reported to be able to differentiate not only into mesoderm-type cells such as osteoblasts, chondrocytes, adipocytes, but also into other cells of non-mesoderm lineages, such as neurocytes, hepatocytes, etc.
- To transplant the RPE to the sub-retinal space is one of the methods for overcoming vision loss. However, RPE for transplantation is poor supply for demand in the process, therefore, method to obtaining the RPE is still restrictive.
- We introduced to investigate the effect and potential of 3D co-culture of BMSCs and RPE on the differentiation of BMSCs into RPE-like cells to obtain a sufficient number of cells for transplantation.

Culture of ARPE-19 Cells

- ARPE-19 was used and purchased from ATCC (American Type Culture Collection, Manassas, Virginia, USA).
- The cells were cultured in DMEM/F12 nutrient mixture supplemented with 10% FBS and 1% antibiotics.
- These cells were suspended in culture plate and incubated at 37°C in humidified atmosphere of 5% CO_2. The medium was changed every 3 days through the experiment.

Differentiation Design of RPE-like Cells

- There are 2 control groups and 2 experimental groups. The control groups are cultured only RPE (Control I) and only

BMSCs (Control II). Experimental groups are that BMSCs are cultured with medium in plate cultured the RPE (Group I) and 3D co-cultured BMSCs using cell culture insert (Group II).

- Insert is used to exclude the effect by the physical contact for the mixed co-culture of BMSCs and RPE.
- All groups are cultured in DMEM supplemented 10% FBS and 1% P/S.
- These schematic diagrams are shown in Fig 1.

Analysis for Differentiation of RPE-like Cells *In Vitro*

- Using a phase contrast microscope, the morphologies of the cells were examined at 1, 3, 7 and 14 days to observe the pattern of morphological change of the cells.
- Cytokeratin can be found in epithelial cells and RPE65 is required for the production and change cycle of vitamin A. They were stained by immunocytochemistry.
- RPE65 and RPE specific marker are used for RT-PCR.

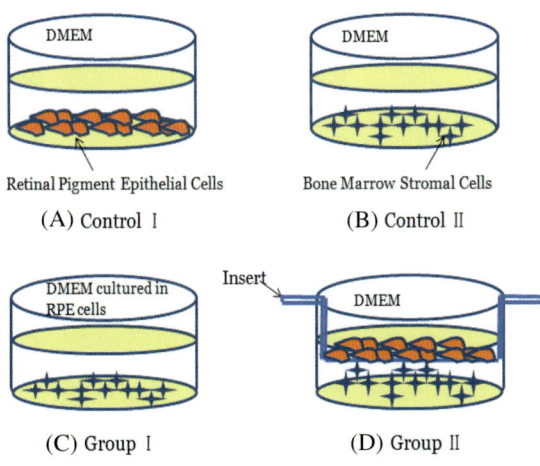

Fig. 1 Schematic diagram of the co-culture models with BMSCs and RPE.

Requirements

DMEM (low glucose), antibiotics (100 unit/mL penicillin and 100 μg/mL streptomycin), HBSS, PBS, trypsin-EDTA, FBS, Ficoll-Paque (specific gravity 1.077 g/mL).

Characterization

- Spindle-shaped cells as characteristic of BMSCs are observed in Control II and cobble stone-shaped cells as retina-specific cells are observed in Control I (Fig. 2).
- BMSCs into RPE were observed on days 7 and 14. The rate of differentiation and proliferation was higher in Group II than in Group I (Fig. 2).
- The rate of differentiation in Group I was slower than for cells in Group II. It might be believed that the rate of effective differentiation in Group I was slower due to the lack of continuous interaction with RPE. BMSCs in Group II can be effectively differentiated into RPE by the various secretions such as cytokine and RPE65 from the RPE and the continuous interaction with RPE (Figs. 3 and 4).

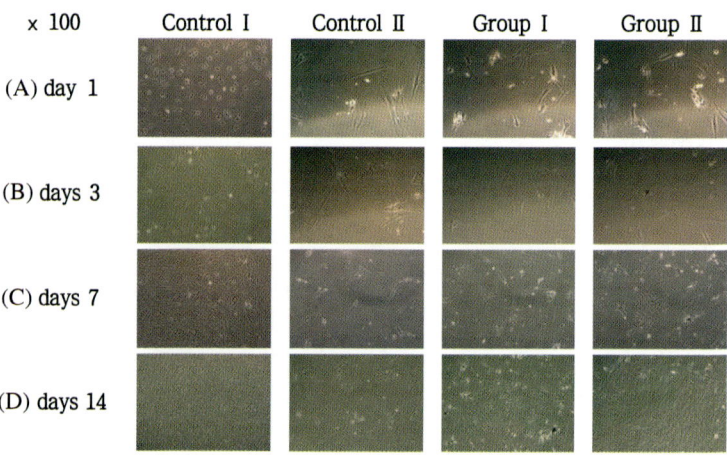

Fig. 2 Morphology of BMSCs analyzed by light microscopic after (A) 1, (B) 3, (C) 7 and (D) 14 days.[1]

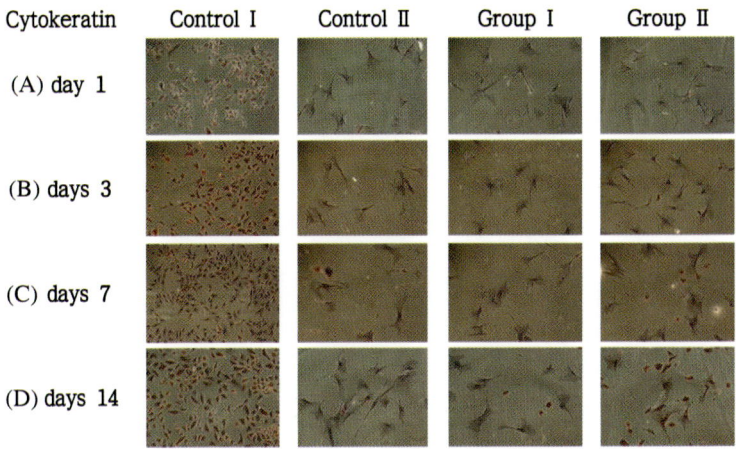

Fig. 3 Immunocytochemical stain with cytokeratin as RPE-specific marker after (A) 1, (B) 3, (C) 7 and (D) 14 days (magnification ×100).[1]

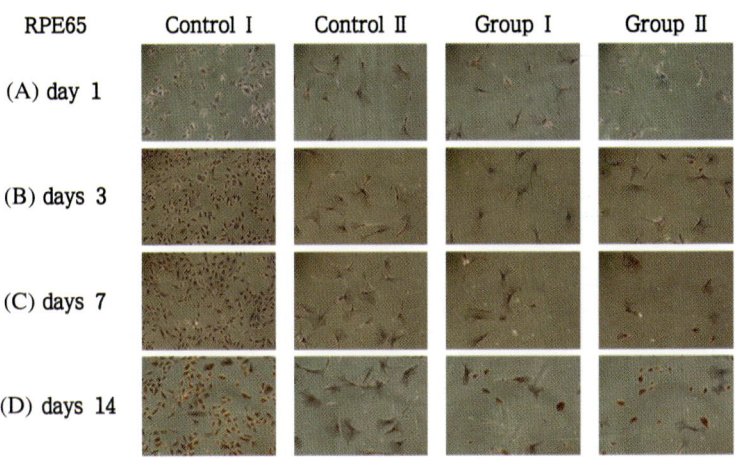

Fig. 4 Immunocytochemical stain with anti-RPE65 as RPE-specific marker after (A) 1, (B) 3, (C) 7 and (D) 14 days (magnification ×100).[1]

• The level of expression of mRNA is shown after standardization into β-actin as a housekeeping gene using RPE65 (Figs. 5 and 6). Figure 5A shows the band indicating the level of expression of β-actin as a housekeeping gene and the expression of β-actin is constant. Also, expression of RPE65 is shown as the band (Fig. 5B).

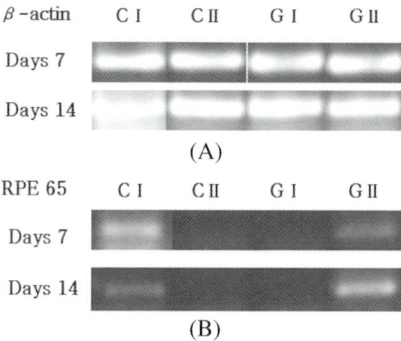

Fig. 5 Gene expression profiles of (A) β-actin (B) RPE65 as analyzed by RT-PCR after 7 and 14 days.[1]

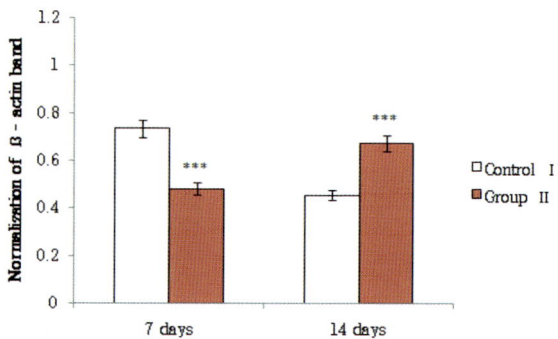

Fig. 6 Expression of mRNA levels in co-culture system after 7 and 14 days by RT-PCR. Normalization of β-actin expression by RPE65 (*** $p < 0.001$).[1]

• These results could suggest that 3D co-culture system may be useful for differentiation of BMSCs into RPE to improve the yield of the RPE efficiently.

Acknowledgments

This research was supported by WCU (R312-0029, KMEST), Bio-industry Technology Development Program (112007-05-1-SB010,

MKFAFF) and Bio & Medical Technology Development Program (2012M3A9C6050204, KMEST).

Reference

1. SJ Cho, SJ Kim, SM Jeong, *et al.* (2011) Differentiation of bone marrow stromal cells to retinal pigment epithelial cells by coculture method using cell culture insert. *Inter J Tissue Regen* **2**(2): 52–58.

R

Protocol of Differentiation of Olfactory Ensheathing Cells from BMSCs by Insert and Conditioned Media System

Jeong Eun Song*, Yun Mi Lee*, Hyeon Yoon*, Chun-Ki Joo†, and Gilson Khang*‡

---

* Dept of BIN Fusion Tech, Polymer Fusion Res Center & Dept of Polymer Nano Sci Tech, Chonbuk National Univ, 567 Baekje-daero, Jeonju 561-756.
† Department of Ophthalmology and Visual Science, College of Medicine, The Catholic University of Korea, Gangnam St. Mary Hospital 505 Banpo-dong, Seocho-gu, Seoul 137-701.

Background

- Olfactory ensheathing cell (OEC) transplantation is a critical and potential therapy for spinal cord injury (SCI).
- BMSCs contain mesenchymal stem cells and progenitor cells. BMSCs can be differentiated into various cell types, including muscle and brain cells.
- This method involves co-culture approach systems using BMSCs (as a source of stem cells) for the differentiation into OECs; OECs and BMSCs were cultured as negative control, respectively, for comparison with differentiation and non-differentiation.
- The experimental groups were designed as follows. In case of group I, the cultured OECs were transferred on the transwell in the 6-well cell culture plate and BMSCs were transferred on the bottom of 6-well cell culture plate. The two cells were co-cultured using the OEC-derived conditioned medium and another case (group II), the BMSCs were cultured on the cell culture plate with OEC-derived conditioned medium. The BMSCs of group II were cultured without OECs for comparison to group I.

Preparation and Culture of OECs[1,2]

- The OECs are isolated from Fischer rats (Japan SLC Inc., Japan).
- Briefly, the olfactory nerve layer is peeled away from the rest of the olfactory bulb without capillary vessels, and then washed 2 times with PBS. For separation of each cell, the olfactory nerve layer is treated with 0.1% collagenase and separated OECs are incubated at 37°C for 30 min.
- For stabilization of cells, the cells are suspended and cultured on the uncoated flask for 18 hr. After incubation, these cells are cultured again for 36 hr with same conditions. And then the cells are seeded on the pre-coated flask with poly(L-lysine) (PLL, 0.1 mg/mL).
- For proliferation of stabilized cells (OECs), the cells are suspended in DMEM supplemented with 10% FBS and 1% PS, 2 μM forskoline and 20 μg/mL bovine pituitary extract (BPE).

- The cells are seeded on the T75 flask at 1×10^5 cells/cm². The medium was changed every 3 days throughout the studies.
- Cultured cells (passage, Fig. 1) are rinsed thoroughly with PBS and detached from flask by trypsin and cultured for experiments.

Culture Methods of rBMSCs

- The femurs (or tibias) are isolated from Fischer rat legs and then washed with PBS. After cutting the tibias, the marrow cavity is flushed with 1 ml PBS using 26G syringe for collection of bone marrow. The flushed bulk bone marrow is spun down in the Percoll cushion solution for 5 min at 2000 rpm. After centrifugation, cell layer in the cushion solution has bone marrow. This bone marrow is spun down again for 10 min at 2500 rpm.
- The collected BMSCs (density of 10^3–10^4 cell/cm²) are cultured at 37°C and 5% CO_2 with DMEM including 10% FBS and 1% antibiotics in culture flask.
- At 3 days after culture, remaining non-adherent hematopoietic cells are removed and washed with PBS including antibiotics. During the incubation, morphology of BMSCs represents adherent spindle-shaped. The medium is changed every 2–3 days during the experiment.
- The sub-culture is carried out when these primary BMSCs reach 80–90% of confluence and these BMSCs (Fig. 2) are used at passage 2 or 3.

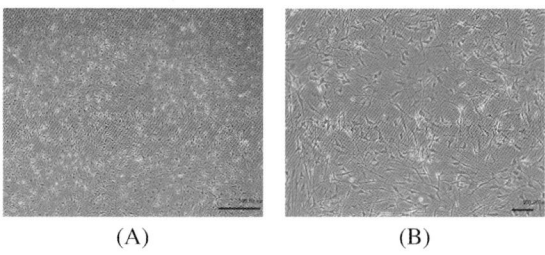

| (A) | (B) |

Fig. 1   Inverted microscope picture of OECs. (A) ×40 and (B) ×100.[1]

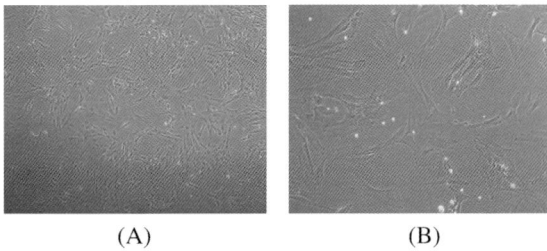

(A)   (B)

Fig. 2   Inverted microscope picture of BMSCs. (A) ×40 and (B) ×100.[1]

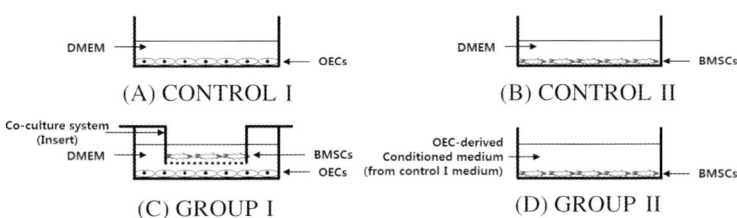

(A) CONTROL I   (B) CONTROL II

(C) GROUP I   (D) GROUP II

Fig. 3   Co-culture model of BMSCs with OECs. (A) Control I (OECs), (B) Control II (BMSCs), (C) Group I (OECs + BMSCs), and (D) Group II (OECs conditioned media + BMSCs).[1]

Co-culture System

- The experimental group I is designed so that OECs are transferred on transwell and co-cultured with BMSCs attached on 6 well bottoms (Fig. 3) [1].
- In another experimental group II, BMSCs are cultured on the flask using OEC-derived conditioned medium. The cells of these experimental groups are fixed at 3, 7, 14, and 21 days after co-culture for characterization.

Characterization

- The expressions of GFAP and P75 are characterized by immunocytochemistry (Figs. 4 and 5).
- RT-PCR is used to evaluate the gene expression of P75, NSE and NF in BMSCs co-cultured with OECs. These results

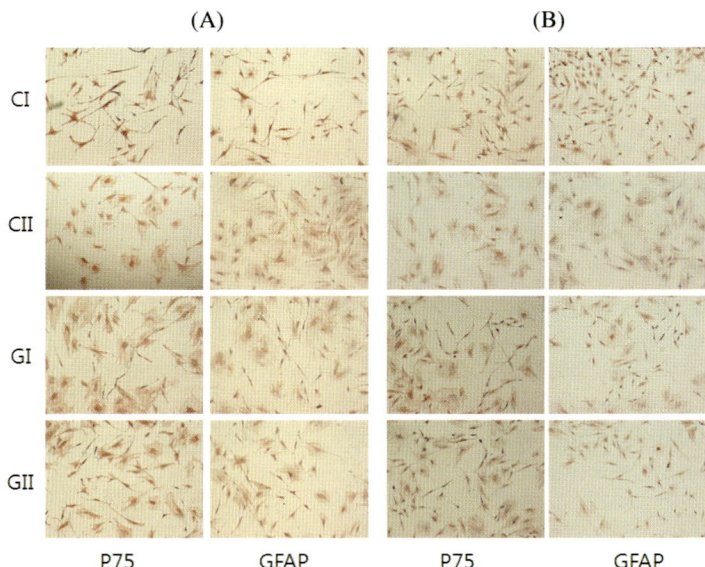

Fig. 4 BMSC images of immunocytochemical staining with P75 and GFAP antibodies (×100). (A) is 3 days and (B) is 7 days after culture.[1]

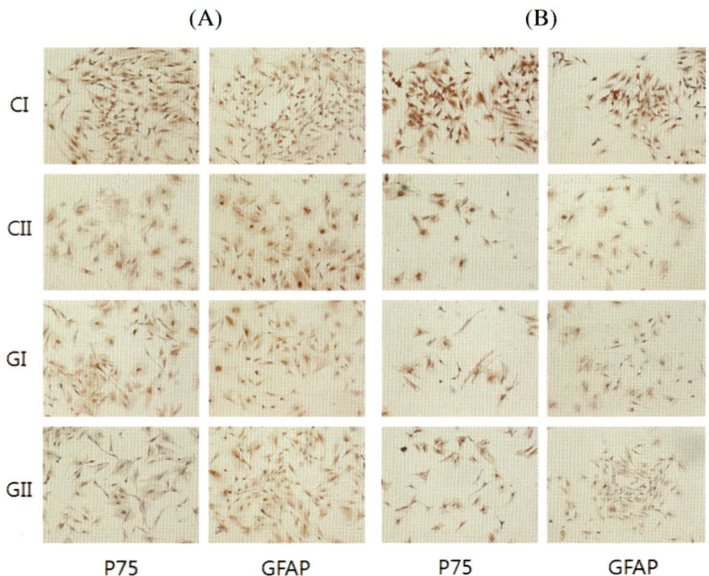

Fig. 5 BMSC images of immunocytochemical staining with P75 and GFAP antibodies (×100). (A) is 14 days and (B) is 21 days after culture.[1]

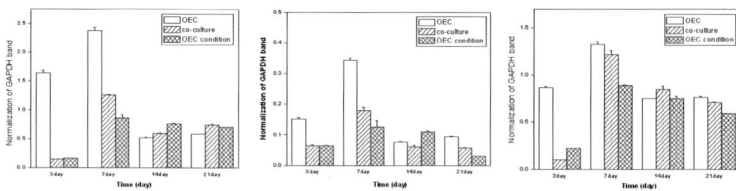

Fig. 6 RT-PCR analysis of gene expression. Normalization by GAPDH band: (A) NF primer, (B) P75 primer and (C) NSE primer.[1]

show that BMSCs can differentiate into OEC-like cells using co-culture system *in vitro* (Fig. 6).

- These findings could be helpful for the development of the cell-based therapeutic strategies for CNS repair.

Acknowledgments

This research was supported by WCU (R31-20029, KMEST), Bio-industry Technology Development Program (112007-05-1-SB010, MKFAFF) and Bio & Medical Technology Development Program (2012M3A9C6050204, KMEST).

References

1. SM Kim, SH Kim, SW Park, *et al.* (2008) Effect of olfactory ensheathing cells on differentiation of bone marrow stem cell. *Tissue Eng Regen Medicine* **5**(1): 117–123.
2. DW Lee, YS Song, CM Kim, *et al.* (2010) Effect of starch-polycaprolactone scaffolds on the attachment, proliferation and phenotypes of olfactory ensheathing cells. *Inter J Tissue Regen* **1**(1): 21–27.

S

Protocol of the Differentiation of BMSC to Corneal Endothelial Cells by Direct and Indirect Co-Culture

Eun Young Kim*, Hyeon Yoon*, Jin San Choi[†], Gilson Khang* and Shay Soker[†]

---

* Dept of BIN Fusion Tech, Polymer Fusion Res Center & Dept of Polymer NanoSci Tech, Chonbuk National Univ, 567 Baekje-daero, Jeonju 561-756.

[†] Wake Forest Institute for Regenerative Medicine, Wake Forest School of Medicine, Medical Center Boulevard, Winston-Salem, NC 27157, USA.

Background

- The corneal endothelium is a thin cell monolayer at the innermost part of the cornea. It helps maintain corneal transparency by regulating stromal hydration using ATPase pumps and serves as a permeable barrier with high metabolic activity.

- Human corneal endothelium has limited self-repair capability *in vivo*. Corneal transplantation is a common procedure performed to improve vision by replacing the opaque or diseased cornea with a clear, healthy donor cornea. However, the worldwide shortage of donor corneas limits transplantation as a means of replacing a deceased patient cornea with a normal functioning donor cornea.

- To overcome the lack of donor corneas, developing suitable scaffold and preparing sufficient corneal endothelial cells is important to regenerate damaged cornea. There are two approaches for regenerating corneal endothelium. One method is to use cultured donor human corneal endothelial cells (CEnC).[1] Another method is to identify, isolate and culture corneal endothelial stem cells or to use other stem cells derived-corneal endothelial-like cells.[2]

- We tried to establish the protocol for the differentiation of BMSCs to secure enough CEnC.

Culturing Methods of CEnCs[1]

- Descemet's membrane including corneal endothelium was stripped from the stroma under microscope.

- CEnC detached from Descemet's membrane using 0.2% collagenase A incubated at 37°C for 40 min.

- Isolated CEnCs were cultured and expended on diameter 100 mm tissue culture plate at 37°C humidified atmosphere containing 5% CO_2 in culture medium containing endothelial growth medium-2 (EGM-2, Clonetics) supplemented with epidermal growth factor (EGF), vascular endothelial growth factor (VEGF), fibroblast growth factor (FGF), insulin-like growth factor (IGF), hydrocortisone, gentamicin, amphotericin-B, and 10% FBS.

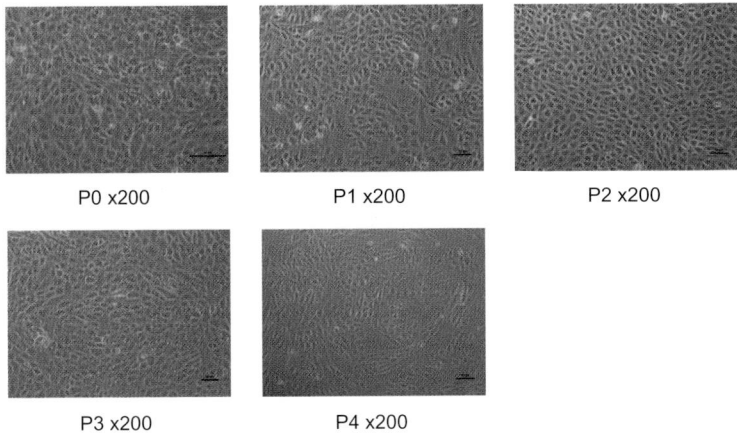

| P0 x200 | P1 x200 | P2 x200 |

| P3 x200 | P4 x200 |

Fig. 1 Morphology of primary culture CEnCs at passage 0 to passage 4 (P: passage, scale bar: 100 μm in magnification ×200).

- Medium was changed every 2 days.
- After 2 weeks of isolation, CEnCs attached to tissue culture plate and reached confluent after about 3 weeks. Confluent CEnCs were subcultured using 0.05% trypsin-EDTA, then reseeded and cultured.
- CEnCs were subcultured until losing their specific morphology whenever CEnCs are reaching confluent. Figure 1 shows cultured CEnCs at each passage 0 to 4.

Characterization of CEnCs

- Analyze gene expression of CEnCs by RT-PCR.
- Express Aquaporin, Collagen type VIII, Na^+/K^+ ATPase, VDAC 2, 3 , NBC 1, and CLCN 3 as specific markers of CEnC as shown in Fig. 2.

Direct Co-Culture of CEnCs and BMSCs

- CEnCs and BMSCs were mixed at 5:5, and 2:8 cultured in EGM-2, DMEM low, and DMEM low with B-27 (Fig. 3).

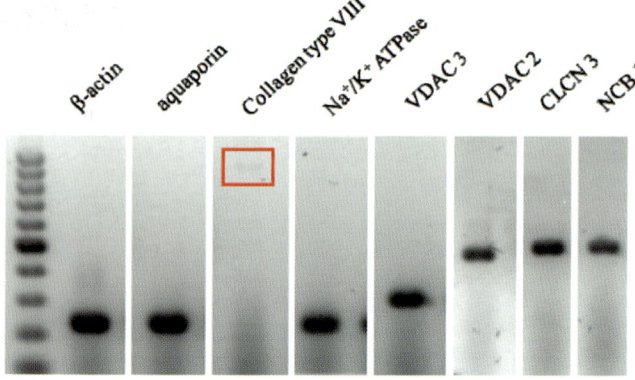

Fig. 2 The gene expression of CEnCs.

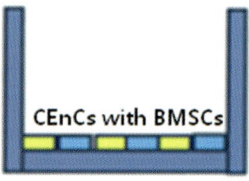

Fig. 3 The schematic illustration of direct co-culture.

- Figure 4 shows direct co-culture morphologic images.
- As time goes by, morphology of BMSCs turned to morphology of CEnCs.
- Comparing diverse medium conditions, changing in EGM-2 shows more compact polygonal morphology and smaller size of turned cells, especially.
- B-27 is an optimized serum substitute developed for low-density plating and long-term viability and growth of hippocampal and other CNS neurons.
- B-27 was added because origin of CEnCs is neural crest.

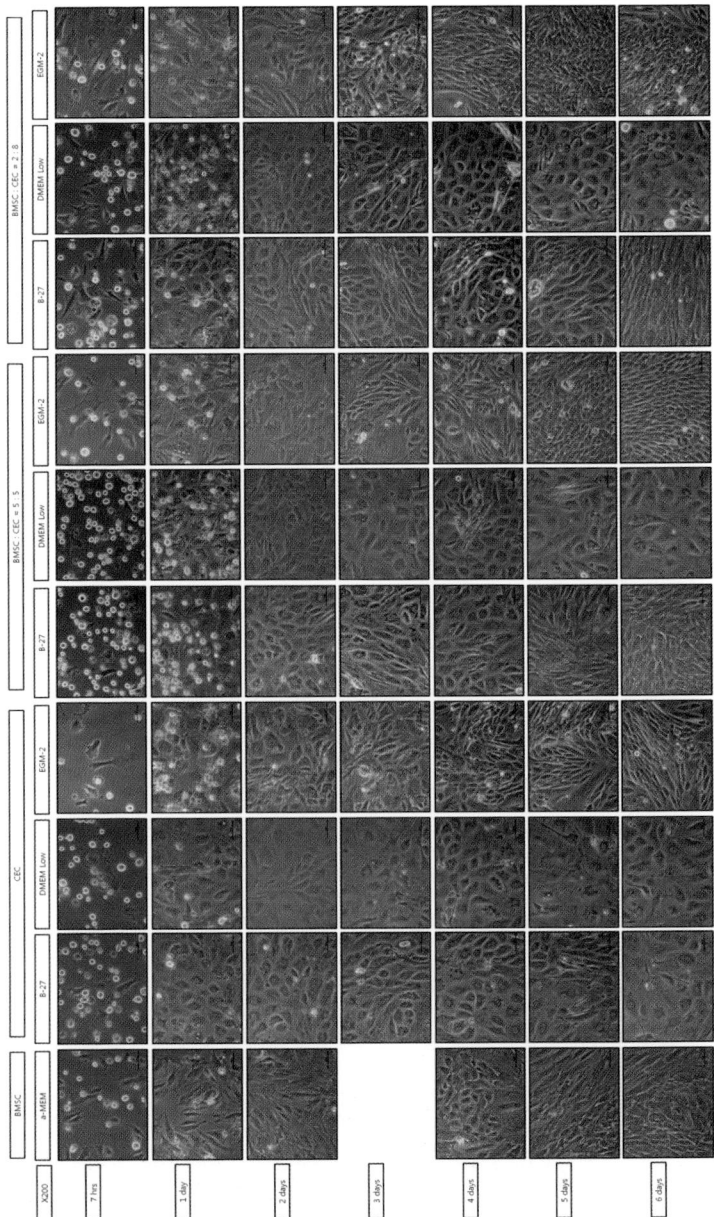

Fig. 4 The morphology of derived-CEnCs at from 7 hr to 6 days after direct co-culture on each condition (magnification ×200).

Analysis for Characterization of Derived CEnCs from BMSCs

- CEnCs and turned cells on each group express Collagen type VIII gene as a specific marker of CEnCs (Fig. 5).
- There is no significance among each medium conditions.
- Identify the derived CEnCs by immunofluorescence using specific markers of CEnCs, Na⁺/K⁺ ATPase and ZO-1.
- Express specific markers of CEnCs on turned cells.
- Figure 6A is the result of IF for Na⁺/K⁺ ATPase and ZO-1 in EGM-2
- Figure 6B is the result of IF for Na⁺/K⁺ ATPase and ZO-1 in DMEM.
- Gene expression of turned cells in EGM-2 is better than in DMEM low.
- Cells in EGM-2 condition have more smaller size and lots of cell number.

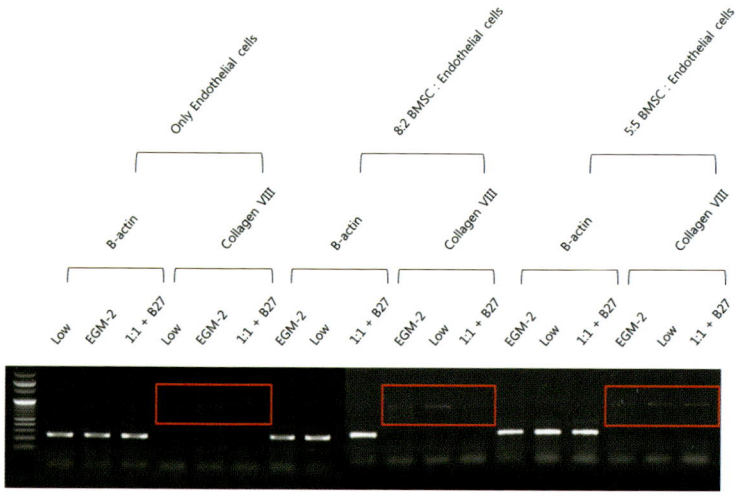

Fig. 5   Collagen type VIII gene expression on turned cell.

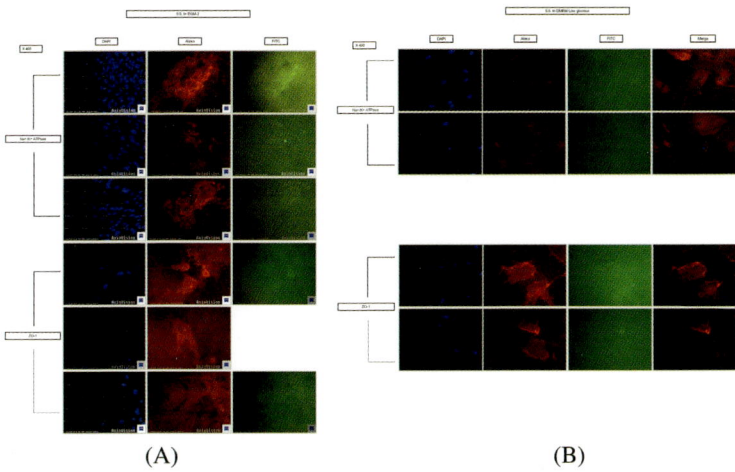

(A) (B)

Fig. 6 ZO-1 and Na$^+$/K$^+$ ATPase gene expression on derived-CEnCs-cultured in (A) EGM-2 or in (B) DMEM low by immunofluorescence (magnification ×400).

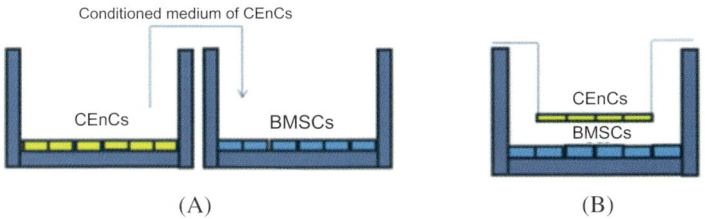

(A) (B)

Fig. 7 The schematic illustration of indirect co-culture of CEnCs and BMSCs using (A) conditioned medium and (B) insert system.

Indirect Co-Culture of CEnCs and BMSCs

- Confirmed morphology from BMSCs to CEnCs using conditioned medium from CEnCs (Fig. 7A) and insert system (Fig. 7B) (Fig. 8).
- Observed polygonal morphology under microscope.

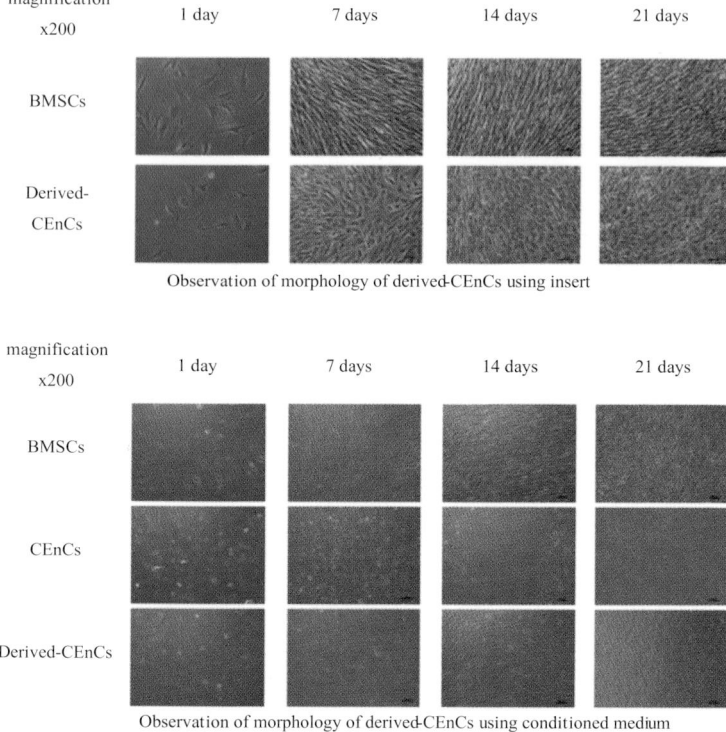

Observation of morphology of derived-CEnCs using insert

Observation of morphology of derived-CEnCs using conditioned medium

Fig. 8 The morphology of differentiated CEnCs from BMSCs using indirect co-culture method (magnification ×200).

Acknowledgments

This research was supported by WCU (R31-20029, KMEST), Bio-industry Technology Development Program (112007-05-1-SB010, MKFAFF) and Bio & Medical Technology Development Program (2012M3A9C6050204, KMEST).

References

1. JS Choi, JK Williams, M Greven, *et al.* (2010) Bioengineering endothelialized neo-corneas using donor-derived corneal endothelial cells and decellularized corneal stroma. *Biomaterials* **31**: 6738–6745.
2. C Shao, Y Fu, W Lu, X Fan. (2011) Bone marrow-derived endothelial progenitor cells: A promising therapeutic alternative for corneal endothelial dysfunction. *Cells Tissues Organs* **193**: 253–263.

Index